Get Through

DCH Clinical

Get Through
DCH Clinical

Andrew Papanikitas BSc (Hons) MA MBBS DCH DPMSA MRCGP
GP Registrar, Aylesbury General Practice Vocational Training Scheme

Helen Goodliffe BSc (Hons) MBBS DCH DRCOG MRCP MRCGP
GP Registrar, Aylesbury General Practice Vocational Training Scheme

Nigel Kennedy MBBS FRCP FRCPCH DCH DRCOG
General Practitioner; Hospital Practitioner (Paediatrics), Stoke Mandeville Hospital, Aylesbury

Published by the Royal Society of Medicine Press Ltd
1 Wimpole Street, London W1G 0AE, UK
Tel: +44 (0)20 7290 2921
Fax: +44 (0)20 7290 2929
E-mail: publishing@rsmpress.co.uk

British Library Cataloguing in Publication Data
A catalogue record for this book is available from the British Library

ISBN: 978-1-85315-764-6

Distribution in Europe and Rest of the World:
Marston Book Services Ltd
PO Box 269
Abingdon
Oxon OX14 4YN, UK
Tel: +44 (0)1235 465500
Fax: +44 (0)1235 465555
Email: direct.order@marston.co.uk

Distribution in USA and Canada:
Royal Society of Medicine Press Ltd
c/o BookMasters Inc
30 Amberwood Parkway
Ashland, OH 44805, USA
Tel: +1 800 247 6553/ +1 800 266 5564
Fax: +1 410 281 6883
Email: order@bookmasters.com

Distribution in Australia and New Zealand:
Elsevier Australia
30–52 Smidmore Street
Marrickville NSW 2204, Australia
Tel: +61 2 9517 8999
Fax: +61 2 9517 2249
Email: service@elsevier.com.au

Phototypeset by MTC Manila
Printed in the UK by Bell & Bain Ltd, Glasgow

Contents

Preface

The Diploma in Child Health (DCH) is a useful exam, not only as evidence of competence in child health, but as part of continuing medical education. We would recommend studying for the exam to any GP or GP-trainee who would like to develop their paediatric knowledge and skills for community practice. Paediatrics, as applied to the community or primary care setting, is not only a compulsory part of nMRCGP and a significant component of the RCGP core curriculum, but a major part of UK general practice. We expect that this book will be a useful aid to revision for the DCH clinical examination. We envisage that some of our material may be of use to GP registrars studying for the nMRCGP clinical skills assessment. We hope that this book will help the reader to understand that though most children are not little adults, they are not little terrors either!

Andrew Papanikitas
Helen Goodliffe
Nigel Kennedy

Acknowledgements

For Mrs Judy Kennedy, Miss Andrea Ogden and Mr Benjamin Bloch, and our families.

Sarah Vasey, Sarah Burrows, Hannah Wessely at the RSM Press and the team at Naughton Project Management.

Dr Craig White, Dr Alix Roberts, Dr Helen Miles, Dr Louisa Barter, Miss Anna Goodliffe, Dr Joseph Papanikitas, Dr Nawal Bahal, Miss Michelle Chan, Dr David, Mr Oliver and Mrs Clare Hughes.

1 Introduction

In an average general practice today, children represent nearly 30% of the list size: 7–10% will be under school age (5 years) and 13% under 15 years. General practitioners (GPs) have responsibility for the care of children with acute and chronic conditions, their development, and preventative and screening programmes for them, including child protection. They must be able to work with the many agencies now involved in the multidisciplinary approach to childcare and to recognize when to call for assistance from the appropriate agency.

The DCH examination

The DCH examination tests candidates in all these spheres of paediatric care and a pass of the examination demonstrates that the doctor has achieved a higher level of competency to carry out their responsibilities to children (www.rcpch.ac.uk/Examinations/DCH). GPs are now able to 'specialize' within primary care as GPwSI (GPs with a special interest), and paediatric medicine lends itself to this type of work.

The DCH examination is organized and set by the Royal College of Paediatrics and Child Health and consists of two parts. Part 1 is a common paper with MRCPCH Part 1A and consists of multiple true/false questions (25), best of five questions (35) and extended matching questions (9). On satisfactory completion of this, DCH candidates then take the Clinical Examination, which from 2006 has been conducted as an OSCE (Objective Structured Clinical Examination) held at centres throughout England and Wales. DCH candidates may sit the DCH Clinical (Part 2) on three occasions only and if unsuccessful are then required to resit Part 1 again.

The OSCE

The OSCE consists of eight clinical stations (www.rcpch.ac.uk/Examinations/DCH/DCH-Clinical-Structure):

1 and 2	Communication skills
3	Structured oral
4	Focused history and management planning
5 and 6	Short clinical
7	Neurodisability
8	Child development

Within these eight stations there are 12 OSCEs. Marks are awarded per OSCE as follows:

Clear pass	12 points
Pass	10 points
Bare pass	8 points
Clear fail	4 points
Unacceptable	0 points

Candidates are currently required to score 120 or more to achieve a pass. They may compensate for lower marks at some OSCEs by scoring higher marks at others, but overall must achieve 120 or greater to pass.

Candidates follow two examination circuits:

Circuit 1: Talking stations (four stations/six OSCEs)

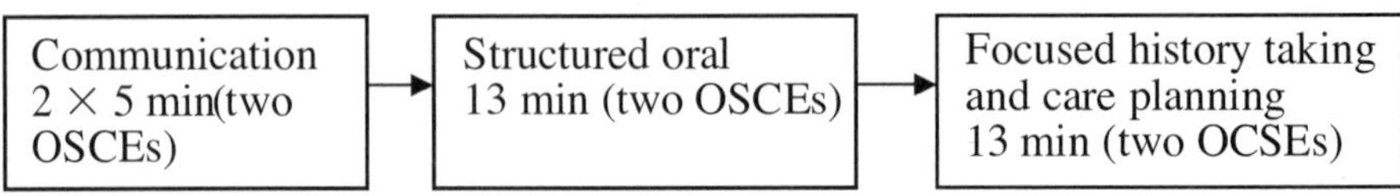

Circuit 2: Clinical stations (four stations/six OSCEs)

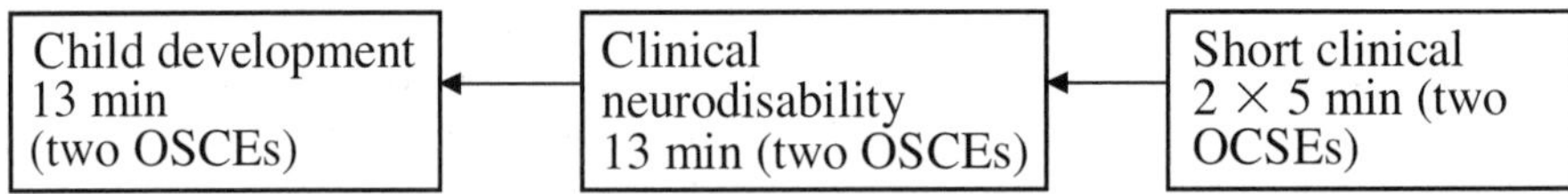

The total time to complete the 12 OSCEs is 90 minutes, with a 3-minute interval between stations. The sequence of OSCEs will vary from centre to centre and may include a break between the two circuits.

Whilst the DCH examination is organized by the RCPCH, DCH examiners are drawn from all areas of paediatric practice. They include hospital and community paediatricians, GPs, child psychiatrists and paediatric surgeons.

Representatives of all these groups play an active part in the formulation of the exam, including exam format and questions, but the examination is focused on a primary-care setting for those working in general practice and community paediatrics.

Detailed knowledge of hospital care is not required, but an understanding of the principles of hospital care is essential for doctors dealing with children in order for them to be able to discuss care/management with parents and carers. Knowledge of common syndromes (e.g. Down's syndrome) is expected, and of rarer but significant conditions is desirable.

The DCH syllabus is available on the RCPCH website (www.rcpch.ac.uk/Examinations/DCH/DCH-Content-Syllabus--General-Info). In addition, guidelines for vision, hearing, language and child surveillance are available on the same website. Anchor statements are available for each type of OSCE station and give clear guidance to candidates on the standards expected of them; in this book, subsequent chapters are preceded by the relevant anchor statement.

Paediatric training recommendation

Regarding paediatric training, it is recommended, but not a prerequisite, that candidates sitting the exam have at least 6 months' hospital experience in paediatrics (www.rcpch.ac.uk/Examinations/DCH/DCH-FAQs; www.rcpch.ac.uk/Examinations/DCH/DCH-How-to-Apply). Hong Kong candidates are required to have 6 months' paediatric experience. Candidates without any paediatric experience are at a significant disadvantage.

What to take into the exam

What to take	What not to take
Stethoscope	Textbooks
Pen torch	Electronic equipment (mobiles and handhelds) should be switched off
Measuring tape	Growth chart and urine dipsticks (provided if needed)
Distraction toy	
Photocard driving licence, passport or hospital identification	

Anchor statement:

	Expected standard	PASS
RAPPORT	Full greeting and introduction Clarifies role and agrees aims and objectives Good eye contact and posture. Perceived to be actively listening (nod, etc.) with verbal and non-verbal cues Appropriate level of confidence, empathetic nature, putting parent/child at ease	Adequately performed but not fully fluent in conducting interview
CLINICAL SKILLS	Appropriate level of confidence Well-structured and systematic examination Correctly identifies and interprets clinical signs and differential diagnosis Suggests appropriate management	Majority of clinical skills demonstrated accurately, eliciting the majority of physical signs correctly Identifies majority of signs correctly May need some prompting and may be some lack of fluency

Short clinical

BARE FAIL	FAIL	UNACCEPTABLE
Incomplete or hesitant greeting and introduction Inadequate identification of role, aims and objectives Poor eye contact and posture. Not perceived to be actively listening (nod, etc.) with verbal and non-verbal cues. Does not show appropriate level of confidence, empathetic nature or putting parent/child at ease.	Significant components omitted or not achieved	Dismissive of parent/child concerns. Fails to put parent or child at ease.
Too many minor errors Examination technique not well structured Non-fluent approach	Misses several important clinical signs Slow, uncertain, unstructured, unsystematic examination	Misses crucial important clinical signs or potentially dangerous interpretation Rough handling of child Disregards child's distress, shyness or modesty

2 The short clinical case

General advice

Always listen carefully to the instructions given to you by the examiner at each station. Failure to carry out the correct task will result in failure to score the relevant marks.

Always introduce yourself to the parent/carer *and* the child, and ask the parent as well as the child for permission to carry out an examination. Ensure that you wash your hands between cases and remember to treat each child with the courtesy and dignity to which they are entitled.

Dealing with a shy, frightened or crying child

Try not to get between the child and their parent(s). However, interacting with the child can generate trust and cooperation. Pre-verbal children often respond to interesting sights and sounds such as a shiny bunch of keys, a rattle or bubbles. Be inventive with what you have available. Attempt to distract them if possible, e.g. by offering to let them hold a toy, playing 'peep-oh' or pulling faces. Let them play with any equipment you may have (within reason!). Older (verbal) children can be challenged, 'I bet you can't open your mouth as wide as mine,' or involved in the examination, 'What sound does your tummy make?'

If a child is clearly distressed, you may need to give them space to calm down and the station may need to be deferred. Examiners should make allowance for this. Children should be treated with respect in any exam, whether undergraduate or postgraduate.

Cardiovascular examination

The most important advice at the outset is to reinforce the need to listen to the examiner's instructions. They may give you a specific task or a more general one to carry out. You must act accordingly or be at risk of losing marks.

- Inspection
- Percussion
- Palpation
- Auscultation

Inspection

- Look at nutritional status – is the child especially small, thin or fat?
- Consider dysmorphic features which may suggest a syndrome, e.g. Down's, Marfan's, Turner's or Noonan's syndromes
- Check for cyanosis:
  - peripheral, e.g. nail beds
  - central, e.g. under tongue
- Check for pallor – anaemia (conjunctiva/mucous membranes)
- Check for plethora – polycythaemia (cyanotic heart disease)
- Check for surgical scars (Fig. 2.1) (ensure that you examine the back and under the arms):
  - left thoracotomy, e.g. patent ductus arteriosus (PDA) ligation, aortic coarctation repair, pulmonary artery banding
  - sternotomy, e.g. complex cardiac surgery
- Fingers:
  - check clubbing, e.g. cyanotic heart disease
  - splinter haemorrhages, e.g. subacute bacterial endocarditis
  - tendon xanthoma, e.g. dyslipidaemia
- Hands:
  - absent radii (VACTERL, a non-random association of abnormalities which may be associated with statin use in the first trimester of pregnancy)
  - absent thumbs (Holt–Oram syndrome – about 75% have heart problems; all have at least one limb abnormality that affects bones in the wrist)

Percussion

Percussion is not often helpful but it may be useful in pericardial effusion. The liver edge may be percussed for hepatomegaly in cardiac failure.

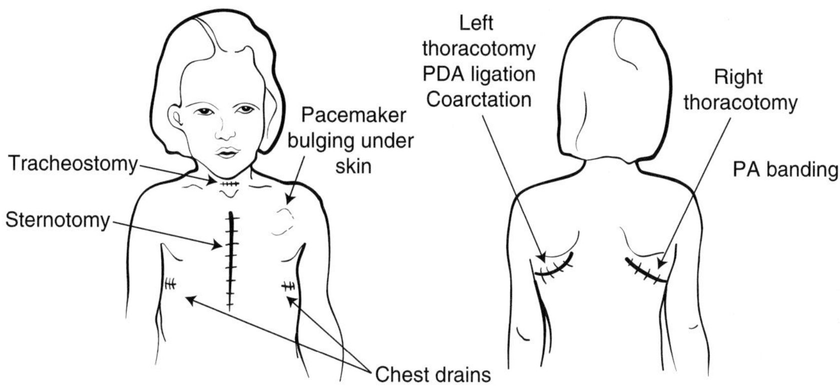

FIGURE 2.1 Surgical scars in children who have had heart or lung surgery.

Palpation

- **General:**
  - check both radial/brachial pulses (brachial often easier to feel)
  - causes of absent brachial/radial pulses:
    - congenital absence
    - previous cardiac surgery, e.g. coarctation of the aorta
    - angioplasty
    - absent/delayed femoral pulse – coarctation
- **Rate:**
  - bradycardia – congenital/complete heart block/beta-blockers
  - tachycardia – anxiety, thyrotoxicosis
- **Rhythm:**
  - sinus arrhythmia (pulse rate decreases on inspiration – a normal finding which is more pronounced in sporty children)
  - irregular: atrial fibrillation (AF) and ectopics (exercise abolishes these)
- **Volume:**
  - decreased volume: shock/hypovolaemia, heart failure or aortic stenosis
  - increased volume (high output states): anaemia, thyrotoxicosis and CO_2 retention
- **Character** (felt at the carotid in the older child or at the brachial artery in the younger child):
  - slowly rising pulse –aortic stenosis (AS)
  - collapsing pulse – aortic incompetence (AI)

- pulsus paradoxus seen in acute asthma and pericardial effusion (very unlikely to be seen in the exam, which uses clinically stable children with clinically stable signs)
- jerky pulse – hypertrophic cardiomyopathy (HCM)

Femoral pulse absent/delayed = coarctation of the aorta

Ask to check BP (the cuff must occlude two-thirds of the upper arm, i.e. be an appropriate size!). Refer to centile charts for age appropriate values.

Apex beat position

4th–5th intercostal space inside mid-clavicular line (MCL). Displacement to left represents cardiomegaly or spinal abnormality, e.g. scoliosis/pectus excavatum. Dextrocardia is where the apex beat is felt on the right side, e.g. Kartagener syndrome, which is characterized by transposition of the internal organs of the body as well as congenital malformation of respiratory cilia with resulting sinusitis and bronchiectasis. So, if you cannot feel an apex beat, always check on the opposite side.

Thrills

- Left parasternal = right ventricular hypertrophy
- Lower left sternal edge = ventricular septal defect
- Upper left sternal edge = pulmonary stenosis
- Suprasternal = aortic stenosis

Type

- Forceful = left ventricular hypertrophy
- Heave = right ventricular hypertrophy (parasternal left sternal border)

Auscultation

Unless instructed otherwise by the examiner, examine all four areas (Fig. 2.2):

1. Aortic – right 2nd intercostal space (ICS)
2. Pulmonary – left 2nd ICS
3. Tricuspid – left lower sternal edge
4. Mitral – left 5th ICS, mid-clavicular line

Hearts sounds

- Murmurs
- Added sounds
- First heart sound – closure of mitral and tricuspid valves

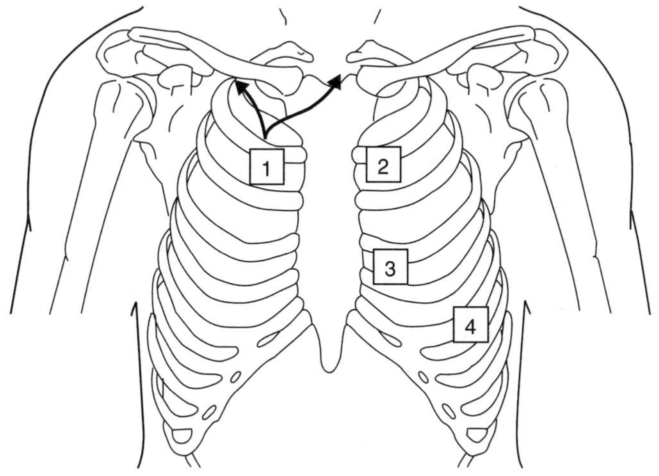

FIGURE 2.2 Auscultation areas.

- Second heart sound – closure of aortic and pulmonary valves. Note physiological split of second heart sound which widens on inspiration. Remember a fixed split second heart sound = atrial septal defect (ASD)

Murmurs

- Loudness is graded 1–6 systolic and 1–4 diastolic
- A palpable thrill represents a murmur > Grade 4
- Site
- Radiation
- Timing, e.g. continuous murmur (machinery) in PDA
- Pitch
- Relationship to posture and respiration

Innocent murmur (benign):

- no symptoms
- systolic
- short
- soft
- normal split P2 (widens on inspiration)

- varies with posture
- normal ECG, chest X-ray and echocardiogram

Normal murmurs:

- benign (see above)
- pulmonary flow–best heard at L 2nd ICS
- venous hum–best heard above clavicle
- neonatal peripheral pulmonary artery stenosis

Pathological murmurs (systolic):

- ventricular septal defect – lower left sternal edge
- pulmonary stenosis – upper left sternal edge
- atrial septal defect – upper left sternal edge, fixed split P2
- aortic stenosis – 2nd right upper ICS (possible by bicuspid aortic valve)
- coarctation of the aorta – systolic murmur radiating to the back
- mitral incompetence – mitral area
- mitral valve prolapse – mitral area

Cardiovascular short cases

Cyanotic congenital heart disease

One-third of congenital cardiac defects:

- Transposition of great vessels
- Fallot tetralogy
- Pulmonary atresia
- Shunt R→ L

These children are far more likely to be seen in an exam post-operation, on the basis that clinically unstable children will not be used in OSCEs.

Acyanotic congenital heart disease

Two-thirds of congenital cardiac defects:

- VSD
- ASD
- PDA
- PS
- AS
- Coarctation
- Shunt L→R

Respiratory examination

It is extremely important to listen to the examiner's instructions. Only undress the child to the waist after asking the parents' and child's permission. This is particularly important with adolescent girls.

- Inspection
- Percussion
- Palpation
- Auscultation

Inspection

- General nutritional status
- Check for respiratory aids and devices, e.g. spacers, peak flow, supplemental oxygen
- Check for clubbing (cystic fibrosis, congenital cyanotic heart disease)
- Check for cyanosis (respiratory and cardiac causes)
- Listen for stridor, both inspiratory and expiratory, and wheeze
- Check skin, e.g. eczema, or possibility of asthma/atopy

Chest shape

- Deformity, e.g. scoliosis
- Asymmetry, e.g. fibrosis/hypoplasia
- Hyperinflation, e.g. asthma
- Harrison's sulcus – association with chronic respiratory distress (surgery may reverse this sign)
- Absent pectoralis major – Poland syndrome (an absent or underdeveloped pectoralis on one side of the body and webbing of the fingers of the ipsilateral hand)
- Pectus excavatum (hollow chest)
- Pectus carinatum (pigeon chest)

Chest scars

Such as chest drain scars or a tracheostomy scar (see Fig. 2.1).

Accessory muscles

- Nasal flaring, intercostal or subcostal recession
- Use of abdominal muscles

Respiratory rate

- Infant: 20–40/min
- 5-year-old: 15–25/min
- 10-year-old: 15–20/min

Cough

- Barking = laryngeal
- Moist = lower respiratory tract infection
- Paroxysmal = pertussis

Palpation

- Check position of trachea – deviation with effusion and pneumothorax
- Check chest expansion by circling hands around the child's chest, placing thumbs at level of the nipples – is it symmetrical or reduced? (> 4 cm is normal)

Tactile vocal fremitus (TVF)

Place the palm of the hand on the upper chest wall and ask the child to say 99, comparing left to right. Increased TVF occurs in consolidation and is reduced or absent with collapse and/or pleural thickening and/or effusion.

Percussion

This is useful to assess the presence of hyperinflation, i.e. with increased resonance, to check liver size or determine presence of consolidation, effusion or collapsed lung.

- Resonant – normal
- Hyperresonant – pneumothorax
- Dull – consolidation and fibrosis
- Stony dull – pleural effusion

Auscultation

- **Normal:** vesicular sounds
- **Abnormal:**
  - bronchial: harsh sounds, expiratory phase same length as inspiration
  - breaths diminished or absent suggest no air or fluid
  - expiratory wheeze: asthma/bronchiolitis foreign body

- fine crepitations: fibrosis/pulmonary oedema
- coarse crepitations: infective/bronchiectasis
- pleural rub: only with dry pleurisy, lost with effusion

Vocal resonance

- Ask the child to say 99 whilst listening over both lung fields
- Increased with consolidation
- Lost or reduced with fluid/no air
- Listen for whispering pectoriloquy or aegophony which can be heard just above a pleural effusion

Abdominal examination

Introduce yourself to the parents and child and remember to ask permission to examine the child. Modesty must be observed using a blanket. Remember warm hands are helpful for examination.

Listen to the instructions from the examiner and only carry out what is asked of you, e.g. 'Please examine for a spleen' or 'Please examine the abdomen'.

- Inspection
- Palpation
- Percussion
- Auscultation

Check for:

- **Face and mucous membrane:** anaemia (mucous membranes), jaundice (sclera), spider naevi, mouth for pigmentation – Peutz–Jegher/Addison or angioma (hereditary haemorrhagic telangiectasia)
- **Dysmorphic features:** mucopolysaccharidoses
- **Chronic liver disease:** stigmata – palmar erythema, clubbing, leuconychia, koilonychia
- **Tongue:** Down's (pseudomacroglossia), Beckwith–Wiedemann (macroglossia)

Causes of clubbing in children

- Cystic fibrosis (CF)
- Inflammatory bowel disease (Crohn's disease/colitis)
- Congenital cyanotic heart disease

Abdominal inspection

Scars, e.g. stoma (ileostomy/colostomy), splenectomy/appendicectomy, major surgery, laparoscopy (Fig. 2.3).

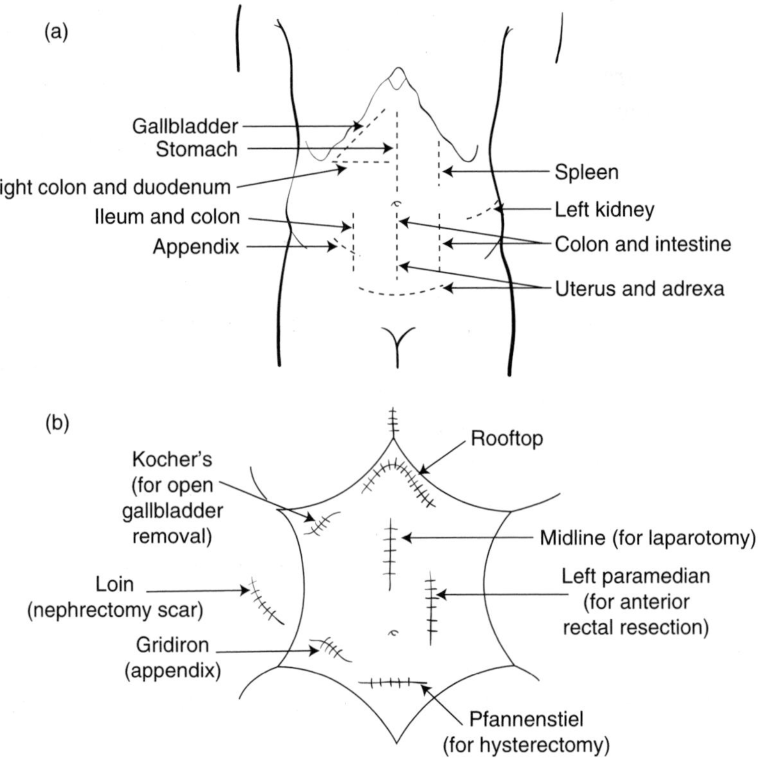

FIGURE 2.3 (a) Abdominal scar identification. (b) Abdominal incisions and their names.

Striae may be present. A hernia may be visible in the abdominal wall or as a mass on inspection of the scrotum, e.g. hydrocoele and hernia.

Abdominal distension

- Fat
- Faeces – constipation/Hirschsprung's
- Flatus – aerophagy/malabsorption
- Fluid – ascites
- 'Flipping big mass' or fetus (it is highly unlikely that a pregnant child would consent to be a DCH examination patient)

Palpation

First explain to the child and parent what you are going to do, and be very gentle. Examination consists of both superficial and deep palpation of all four quadrants in turn. If tenderness is elicited, try to localize it and check for guarding or rebound. Watch the child's face at all times for any sign of discomfort. Distract younger children with comments such as, 'Can we feel lunch in your tummy?'

Individual organs

- **Liver** – start the examination in the right iliac fossa (RIF) and work up towards the right costal margin. A palpable liver in children is not unusual up to 2 cm. Percuss the upper border of the liver as well as the lower to exclude hyperinflation as a cause of hepatomegaly.
- **Spleen** – start the examination in the RIF and work up towards the left upper quadrant. To feel the spleen you may need to turn the child onto their right side and ask them to take a deep breath. Feel for the splenic notch. This is not a consistent finding in children.
- **Kidney** – examine bimanually in order to palpate for a kidney. An enlarged kidney may be ballotable.

Abdominal masses

Try to identify site, size and consistency. Check for mobility and tenderness.

Percussion/auscultation

- Fluid, i.e. ascites – test for shifting dullness
- Mass/organomegaly
- Bowel sounds
- Renal bruits (in neurofibromatosis may have hypertension due to renal artery stenosis)
- Testes – do not routinely examine; only if requested by examiner

Lastly, 'I would like to conclude my examination by…'

- Examining the external genitalia
- Plotting height and weight on a growth chart
- Dipping the urine for blood, protein, leucocytes and nitrites

Cerebellar examination

A disturbance of cerebellar function leads to a lack of coordination of movement. The following signs are indicative of cerebellar dysfunction:

- Scanning dysarthria
- Nystagmus
- Dysdiadochokinesis
- Intention tremor
- Past pointing dysmetria
- Ataxic gait (poor heel-to-toe walking)
- Romberg's sign, a tendency to sway or fall while standing upright with the feet together. This usually indicates an inner ear problem or a failure of proprioception

Gait

- **Normal variations:**
  - toe walking (tiptoeing) – 'little ballerina syndrome'. This may also be an early indicator of myopathy and spastic diplegia (cerebral palsy)
  - in-toeing and out-toeing
  - bow legs (Genu varum)
  - knock knees (Genu vagum). Pathological causes include rickets and Blount disease
- **Abnormal gaits** (Fig. 2.4):
  - broad based gait is often associated with cerebral palsy
  - waddling gait is often associated with untreated developmental dysplasia of the hip and Duchenne's muscular dystrophy
  - hemiplegic gait
  - spastic diplegia
  - ataxic gait (cerebellar dysfunction)
  - athetoid gait
  - limp (antalgic gait)

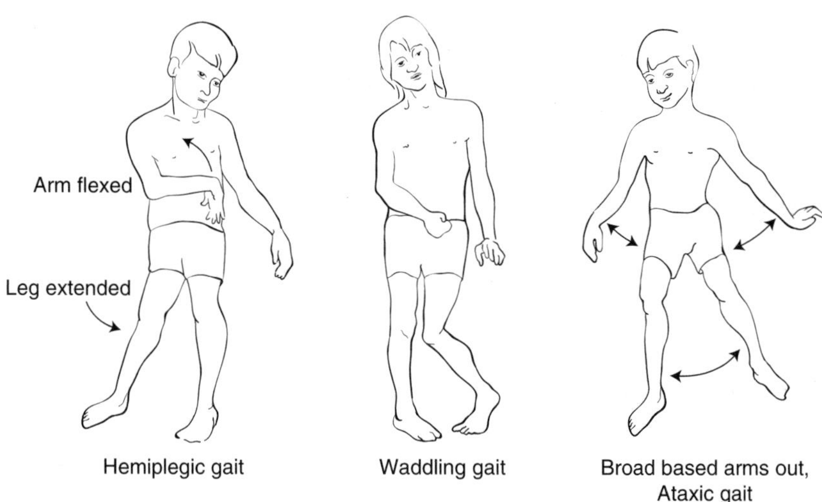

FIGURE 2.4 Abnormal gaits.

Thyroid examination (see box on page 20)

Inspection

Look for goitre and also examine neck for thyroglossal cyst (protrusion of tongue causes cyst to move). Also look for ectopic thyroid (back of tongue).

Palpation

Examine from behind to feel the neck: swallowing with water will help. Remember a retrosternal thyroid may cause palpable tracheal deviation in the suprasternal notch.

Move on to assess thyroid status.

Common syndromes

Neurocutaneous syndromes

- Neurofibromatosis (see Chapter 3)
- Tuberous sclerosis (see Chapter 3)

Hypothyroidism	Hyperthyroidism
Obesity	Sweating
Short stature	Increased appetite
Puffy eyes	Weight loss
Dry skin	Goitre and/or bruit
Slow pulse	Fine tremor
Cold intolerance	Warm moist palms
Delayed relaxation of tendon reflexes	Exophthalmos
	Lid lag and lid retraction
	Ophthalmoplegia
	CVS – high output state, ejection systolic murmur, hypertension
	Proximal myopathy

Sturge–Weber syndrome

- Associated with epilepsy, learning disabilities and hemiplegia
- Sporadic condition
- Haemangiomatous facial lesions in the 5th cranial nerve distribution associated with haemangiomata of the meninges. This always affects the ophthalmic division and often the maxillary and mandibular divisions as well

Skull X-ray shows cerebral calcification. Differential diagnosis of cerebral calcification includes:

- Arteriovenous malformations
- Toxoplasmosis
- Cytomegalovirus
- Glioma/astrocytoma
- Craniopharyngioma

Lysosomal enzyme storage disorders

- Mucopolysaccharidoses (Hunter and Hurler syndromes)
- Lipid storage disorders: Tay–Sachs, Gaucher, Niemann–Pick

Hurler's syndrome

Autosomal recessive disorder. Developmental delay from 6–12 months. Features include:

- Clouding of cornea
- Glaucoma
- Coarse facial features
- Large tongue
- Excess hair
- Bones – thick skull, kyphosis in thoracolumbar region
- Heart – valvular lesions and heart failure
- Neurodevelopment – regressive development
- Hepatosplenomegaly

Hunter's syndrome

X-linked recessive disorder. No cornea clouding and less severe changes.

Chromosomal disorders

Down's syndrome (trisomy 21)

This is the commonest chromosomal abnormality seen in practice. The clinical features and bio-psycho-social implications are considered more fully in Chapters 3 and 7. Down's syndrome can affect several organ systems and the child commonly has characteristic dysmorphic features. Children with Down's syndrome frequently participate in paediatric examinations. *Know this condition and its associated features.*

Turner's syndrome (Fig. 2.5)

Chromosomes: XO. Incidence 1/2000–2500.

Noonan's syndrome

(Male version of Turner's but is now known to occur in both sexes.) Incidence 1/2000.

- Downward sloping palpebral fissures
- High arched palate
- Webbing of neck
- Short stature
- Pectus excavatum
- Right heart abnormalities including atrial septal defect and pulmonary stenosis

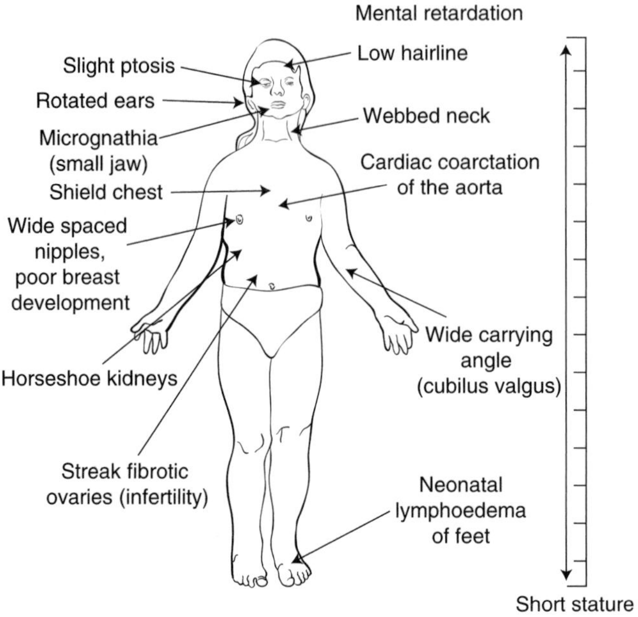

FIGURE 2.5 Features of Turner's syndrome.

Williams syndrome

- Supravalvular aortic stenosis
- Learning disabilities
- Notable feature: transient neonatal hypercalcaemia

Prader–Willi syndrome

Incidence 1/10 000. Deletion of the long arm of chromosome 15.

- Hypotonia in neonates
- Later development of obesity
- Hypogonadism
- Developmental delay
- Small hands and feet

- Short stature
- Scoliosis

Further reading

Papanikitas A, Bahal N, Chan M. *Get Through Clinical Finals: A Toolkit for OSCEs*. London: RSM Press, 2006: p. 211–2, 220.

Anchor statement:

	Expected standard/ CLEAR PASS	PASS
PART A: RAPPORT	Full greeting and introduction Clarifies role and agrees aims and objectives Good eye contact and posture. Perceived to be actively listening (nod, etc.) with verbal and non-verbal cues Appropriate level of confidence, empathetic nature, putting parent/child at ease	Adequately performed but not fully fluent in conducting interview
PART A: CLINICAL SKILLS	Appropriate level of confidence Well-structured and systematic examination Correctly identifies and interprets clinical signs and differential diagnosis Suggests appropriate management	Majority of clinical skills demonstrated accurately eliciting the majority of physical signs correctly Identifies majority of signs correctly May need some prompting and may be some lack of fluency
PART B: SUMMARY, MANAGEMENT PLANNING AND CLOSURE	Invites further questions Summarizes Gives accurate information Explores options for management Provides appropriate further contact information Refers to other agencies	Summarizes most of the important points and suggests **best** management strategy Provides some information about other services and future plan Deals with uncertainty in diagnosis or management

Neurodisability

BARE FAIL	CLEAR FAIL	UNACCEPTABLE
Incomplete or hesitant greeting and introduction Inadequate identification of role, aims and objectives Poor eye contact and posture. Not perceived to be actively listening (nod etc.) with verbal and non-verbal cues Does not show appropriate level of confidence, empathetic nature or putting parent/child at ease	Significant components omitted or not achieved	Dismissive of parent/child concerns Fails to put parent or child at ease
Too many minor errors Examination technique not well structured Non-fluent approach	Misses several important clinical signs. Slow, uncertain, unstructured, unsystematic examination	Misses crucial important clinical signs or potentially dangerous interpretation Rough handling of child Disregards child's distress or shyness or modesty
Incomplete summary of problems and inadequately planned management Does not relate management to child's/parents' needs or concerns Inadequate attempt to determine child's/parents' understanding	Poor summary Patient unsure of future plans. Poor discussion of management options Poor exploration of parents' or child's views or desires about treatment Poor use of referral to other agencies	Abrupt ending. Inaccurate information given. Lack of regard for safe, ethical and effective treatments Poor arrangements for future contact

3 Neurodisability cases

You will be asked to examine a child with a neurodisability. Try to perform a relevant neurological examination and then look at associated features. Try to adopt a holistic approach; looking at the whole child, considering mobility aids, nutrition and other impairments such as hearing and vision. The examiner may direct you to particular aspects of the examination. This station is 13 minutes long. The examination should take approximately 8 minutes, leaving 5 minutes for discussion with the examiner (www.rcpch.ac.uk/Examinations/DCH/DCH-Clinical-Structure).

Practice your approach to examining a child in a wheelchair so that you appear confident in the exam. *Never* make assumptions about a child's intellectual ability from their appearance.

Sometimes the examiner will direct you to ask some initial questions. It is important to direct these to both the child and the parent, and to include those about the child's schooling.

Read the syllabus (www.rcpch.ac.uk/Examinations/DCH/DCH-Content-Syllabus--General-Info) and think about the following topics:

- Assessment and long-term management of children with disabling conditions
- Services available in a district to help children identified with motor, sensory, educational and emotional disability
- Genetic counselling

You will be marked on your rapport, including your greeting, body language, empathy and ability to put the parent and child at ease, and your communication skills. You will also be marked on performing a confident, systematic examination, the ability to elicit and interpret signs, your diagnosis and suggested management. Marks will be given for discussion, including summarizing the case, discussing management, referral to other agencies and knowing where to direct parents for further information (www.rcpch.ac.uk/Examinations/DCH/DCH-Clinical-Structure).

General approach

Introduce yourself to the child and parent and ask permission of both to examine the child. Put the child at ease – chatting to them will also give you an idea of speech problems/learning difficulties. Offer praise and encouragement to the child at each stage of the examination.

Observation

- Posture/limb alignment
- Wheelchair/specialist seating
- Splints
- Shoe raises
- Any obvious abnormalities with limbs/dysmorphic features

Ask if they are able to walk/transfer to couch. *Watch gait.*

Gait abnormalities (see Fig. 2.4)

- Hemiplegia – if walking, try to elicit more subtle signs of a hemiplegia by asking the child to run or distracting them (e.g. by asking them to count backwards whilst walking)
- Spastic scissoring gait
- Ataxia
- Proximal weakness/waddling gait – to elicit proximal weakness ask the child to stand from sitting in a chair with their arms folded or try to elicit Gower's sign (Fig. 3.1): Gower's positive: cannot stand from lying on their back without using their hands – tend to roll over then walk their hands up their legs

Relevant examination

- **Neurological:**
  - inspection of limbs – scars, contractures, muscle wasting
  - test limbs in an age appropriate way with clear instructions to the child – tone, power, reflexes, coordination, sensation, proprioception

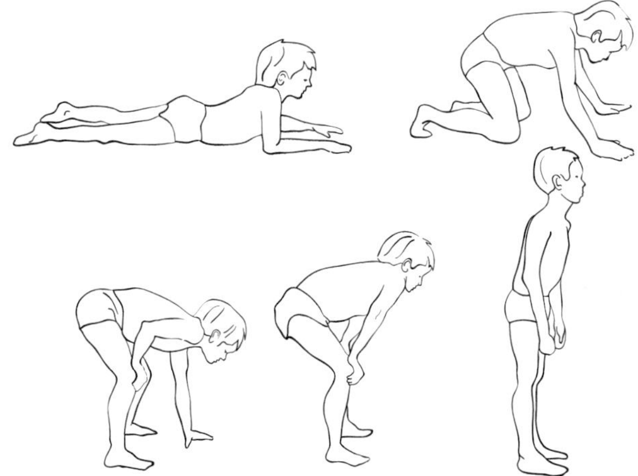

FIGURE 3.1 Gower's sign (seen in Duchenne's muscular dystrophy).

- examine back for scars, scoliosis or evidence of spina bifida
- look at feet/shoes

- **Sensory:**
  - hearing – hearing aids?
  - vision – wearing glasses?
  - squint
  - speech and language, including dentistry/oral care
- **Schooling – statemented?** What support does the child have in school? (For information on the statement of special educational needs, see Chapter 6)
- **Diet:**
  - swallowing OK?
  - hyoscine patch for secretions?
  - PEG (percutaneous endoscopic gastrostomy)
- **Any other medical problems?**

Approach to examining a child in a wheelchair

- Introduce yourself to the child and their parent(s)
- Put them at ease
- Ask permission from child and parent
- Observe
- Ask what the child can do – they may always be in a wheelchair but are able to move arms and legs, or they may just use the wheelchair for trips out of

the house and have a different way of moving around in the home. Can they move to the couch to be examined?

Much of the examination relies on good observation; however, it is possible to examine the limbs in a wheelchair. Practise this so that you are not thrown in the exam if the child is not on the couch.

- Start by observing the limbs, their position/posture, abnormal/involuntary movements
- Look for any splints
- Examine for scars – ask child/parent if there are any hidden scars
- Sit the child forward and look at the back for scars/scoliosis/evidence of spina bifida

Examine the limbs as far as possible:

- Inspection – wasting, contractures, scars, fasciculations
- Tone
- Power
- Reflexes
- Coordination
- Sensation
- In addition, look at the range of movement of the joints (passive and active) and look for contractures

If asked to continue, other relevant parts of the examination may include:

- Looking for hyoscine patches
- Examining PEG site
- Listening to lungs
- Assessing for squint
- Head – circumference, fontanelles, shunts

EXAMPLE CASES

Cerebral palsy

A non-progressive motor disorder caused by brain disease.

What to look for on examination

Inspection

- Wheelchair

- Braces
- Calipers
- Leg/arm splints (ankle foot orthoses)
- Shoe raises
- Pressure care
- Spine abnormality
- Size and shape of skull and fontanelles (microcephaly?, hydrocephalus?)

Face

- Any trouble with swallowing/ excessive saliva? (for which they may be wearing a hyoscine patch)
- Hearing aids
- Glasses
- Squint
- Feeding tubes

Limbs

- Posture
- Ability to sit unaided
- Abnormal movements
- Scars/contractures, e.g. shortened Achilles' tendons
- Tone – increased (clonus – best tested at the ankle, may also have clasp knife spasticity)
- Power – may be decreased
- Reflexes – may be increased
- Sensation – normal
- May have extensor plantars
- Coordination – may have ataxia or reduced control due to weakness

Look at gait

- Try to elicit a subtle weakness by requesting manoeuvres that make it more obvious:
  - running, heel-to-toe walking and walking on tip-toes
  - distracting the child by asking them to recite their address or count backwards whilst walking
- May have a stiff-legged, 'scissored' gait
- May have a broad-based ataxic gait
- May have a stiff leg that is swung round
- Look at the upper limbs when they are walking – ?loss of natural arm swing, one arm flexed, hand making a fist

Cerebral palsy in a small child

- Look for hand preference – babies should not show hand preference before the age of 1 year
- Look for scissoring of the legs when the child is lying on their back/lifted

Describe the pattern of neurology you find:

- Hemiplegia
- Quadriplegia
- Diplegia
- Monoplegia
- Ataxia
- Athetoid/dyskinetic
- Spastic

What other medical problems may the child have?

- Deafness
- Visual problems
- Epilepsy
- Contractures
- Dislocation of the hip
- Scoliosis
- Poor lung function/recurrent chest infections
- Poor coordination/ataxia
- Swallowing difficulties
- Reflux
- Nutritional deficiency
- Pooling of saliva/poor dentition
- Learning disabilities
- Incontinence
- Constipation
- Problems with pressure areas

Multiple problems – therefore the child should be managed by a multidisciplinary team. The team may include: community paediatrician GP, physiotherapist, occupational therapist, speech therapist, dietician, gastroenterologist, orthopaedic surgeon and neurologist.

Other considerations

- Support groups, e.g. www.cerebralpalsyinfo.org and www.scope.org.uk
- Education

- Respite care
- Benefits and financial support
- Mobility aids
- Management of hearing and vision problems

Types of cerebral palsy

- **Quadriplegia** – all four limbs affected
- **Hemiplegia** – involvement of the right or left arm and leg
- **Diplegia** – involvement of both legs more than the arms

These may be:

- **Spastic** – increased tone which may affect most movements, or just a particular muscle group or limb. Although the initial insult does not progress, the spasticity may worsen with time. Spastic cerebral palsy results from damage to the motor area of the cerebral cortex
- **Ataxic** – poor coordination, hypotonia, tremor and other cerebellar signs, such as nystagmus. Truncal ataxia and a wide-based gait may be observed. Ataxic cerebral palsy results from damage to the cerebellum
- **Dyskinetic/athetoid** – athetosis describes the constant writhing movements that result from a lack of control of movement. These children may also have difficulty with their speech. Caused by damage to the basal ganglia.
- **Mixed picture**

What is the aetiology?

Cerebral palsy is caused by prenatal, perinatal or postnatal damage to the developing brain (most cases are thought to be due to an insult in utero). The damage to the developing brain, e.g. the motor cortex, is a one-off insult and does not progress or worsen with time. However, the signs and symptoms may appear to evolve as the child fails to meet their milestones of increasingly complex motor tasks and as the spasticity may worsen with time.

Causes include*:

- **Prenatal:**
  - developmental brain abnormalities
  - IUGR
  - prematurity – more common in very premature babies
  - congenital infection

*From Lissauer T, Clayden G. Neurological disorders. In: *Illustrated Textbook of Paediatrics*, 2nd edn. London: Mosby, 2001, p. 373.

- **Perinatal:**
  - asphyxia at birth
  - ischaemia, e.g. placental abruption
  - trauma, e.g. forceps delivery

- **Postnatal insults to the still developing brain:**
  - severe infection such as encephalitis/meningitis/cerebral abscess
  - hypoxic brain injury
  - kernicterus – unconjugated bilirubin (fat-soluble) can cross the blood–brain barrier and cause damage to the basal ganglia. Less common now through the careful monitoring of bilirubin levels, exchange transfusions and the decreased incidence of haemolytic disease of the newborn
  - trauma
  - stroke/intracranial haemorrhage
  - recurrent seizures/status epilepticus
  - severe prolonged hypoglycaemia

Further information and support can be found on www.cerebralpalsyinfo.org and www.scope.org.uk.

Examining a child with an appearance suggestive of Down's syndrome

- Introduction, what is the child's name?
- Permission from parent and child to examine
- Stand back and sensitively comment on short stature/facial characteristics
- Examine hands
- Cardiovascular examination
- Abdominal examination
- Motor and development examination
- Hearing and vision

What medical problems may the child have?

- Hearing loss – increased incidence of glue ear (conductive hearing loss) and sensorineural hearing loss
- Hypothyroidism
- Cardiac defects – especially AVSD
- Duodenal atresia
- Umbilical hernia
- Early-onset Alzheimer disease
- Cataract
- Atlantoaxial instability

- Leukaemia
- Male: infertility
- Female: delayed menarche

How would you manage a child with trisomy 21 in your practice?

- **General** – multidisciplinary team, child centred care
- **Medically** – monitoring for hypothyroidism, prompt treatment of infections (upper respiratory/ears), monitoring of cardiac disease
- **Surgically** – referral for correction of cardiac defects, duodenal atresia, hernia repair, grommets for glue ear
- **Schooling** – almost all children will have special educational needs and will have a 'Statement of Special Educational Needs'. The degree of extra support needed is very variable
- **Other issues** - genetic counselling, family counselling and support (support groups such as www.downs-syndrome.org.uk)

Down's syndrome (trisomy 21)

What to look for on examination (Fig. 3.2)

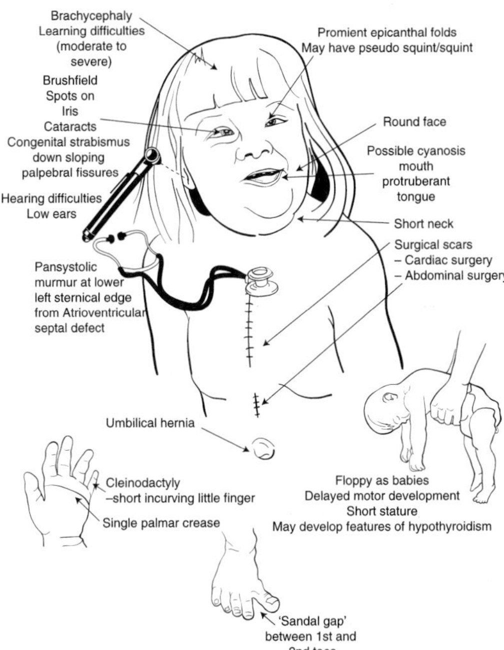

FIGURE 3.2 Features of Down's syndrome.

Genetic counselling

The family want another baby. How would you counsel them about the risks? Explain that most cases of Down's syndrome arise during early development of the baby when the cells are dividing. Sometimes the chromosomes (which contain genes) are not split evenly and by chance the baby gets three copies instead of two copies of a particular chromosome (21). Mostly this is a chance event (95% – non-disjunction during meiosis). However, occasionally one of the parents can carry a faulty copy of a gene (5% of cases; Robertsonian translocation). In these cases the risk of recurrence is higher and both parents should have their chromosomes looked at (karyotyping) to detect this.

The risk of having a child with Down's syndrome increases with maternal age as cell division is more likely to be faulty in the older mother. However, due to the larger number of young women giving birth, the majority of babies with trisomy 21 are born to young mothers. The background risk for all ages is 1/650.

Tests can be offered to screen for Down's syndrome in future pregnancies, including an early scan (nuchal thickness scans) and triple testing (a blood test). These can give an idea of risk but will not indicate whether the baby is definitely affected. Higher risk mothers can go on to have more definitive testing where a sample of cells is collected either by amniocentesis (where a small amount of amniotic fluid from around the baby is collected via a thin needle) or chorionic villus sampling (where a few cells are collected from the placenta). All tests can give false results. The invasive tests do carry a small risk of miscarriage and infection.

Breaking the news that you feel a baby may have Down's syndrome

See Chapter 7. Further information and support can be found at www.downs-syndrome.org.uk.

Tuberous sclerosis

What to look for on examination

- Look at the skin:
  - periungual/subungual fibromas
  - adenoma sebaceum
  - hypomelanotic macules/ash leaf-shaped depigmented patches (which fluoresce under Wood's light)
  - shagreen patch over lumbar spine
- Look for evidence of epilepsy – alert bracelet? gum hypertrophy – phenytoin?

- Look for evidence of renal/cardiac problems – can get renal cysts and tumours such as angiomyolipomas and cardiac rhabdomyomata
- Look for problems with eyesight – can get tumours affecting the eyes, e.g. retinal phakomata
- May also get cerebral astrocytomas

What medical problems may the child have?

- Epilepsy/infantile spasms
- Learning difficulties/developmental delay
- Problems relating to tumours in cardiac, renal and CNS systems, and on retina
- Mostly benign tumours but some malignant potential

How would you investigate a child with tuberous sclerosis?

- Examination of the skin with a Wood's lamp
- Ophthalmological exam
- May need imaging such as a renal US, MRI brain
- May need epilepsy investigations such as an EEG/MRI
- Plot on growth chart
- Screen family
- Genetic testing sometimes used

What sort of management might they need?

- Multidisciplinary team
- Genetics
- Neurology/neurosurgery
- Ophthalmology
- Dermatology/plastics
- Other medical specialities such as cardiology/renal
- Support with learning difficulties – statementing
- Support with epilepsy – education, monitoring, etc.
- Family screening, support and consideration of antenatal testing. Information and support groups for affected families such as the Tuberous Sclerosis Association at www.tuberous-sclerosis.org

What do you know about the inheritance?

Autosomal dominant (20%) or spontaneous mutation (80%).

Duchenne's muscular dystrophy

What to look for on examination

- **General inspection:**
  - wheelchair (by 12 years most children are unable to walk)
  - look for scoliosis
  - look for scars/muscle contractures
  - pseudohypertrophy of calves
- If younger (onset 1–4 years):
  - gait – waddling gait
  - muscle weakness. Positive Gower's sign – ask the child to lie on the floor and stand up. They will tend to walk their hands up their legs due to proximal weakness (see Fig. 3.1)

On examination – muscle weakness.

If time consider examining respiratory and cardiovascular systems:

- Cardiomyopathy
- Respiratory weakness

May have mild learning difficulties.

How would you investigate a child with possible muscular dystrophy?

- Raised serum creatine kinase
- EMG studies
- Muscle biopsy – abnormal dystrophin
- Genetic testing

What do you know about the inheritance?

- X-linked recessive – screen other children in family by testing creatine kinase levels
- Can offer prenatal testing – chorionic villus sampling (CUS)
- Incidence 1/3000 male live births

Becker's muscular dystrophy

A milder form of muscular dystrophy similar to Duchenne's, which tends to present later when the child is about 10–12 years old. Survival is usually to middle age.

*How would you manage a child with muscular dystrophy?**

- Physiotherapy, mobility aids, stretches and splinting to avoid contractures
- Management of scoliosis
- Respiratory support
- Family support and education (e.g. www.muscular-dystrophy.org)
- Family screening/antenatal diagnosis/genetic counselling

Neurofibromatosis

What to look for on examination

- Look at the skin:
  - axillary freckling
  - café-au-lait spots. Light brown patches on the skin (> 5 mm in children, > 15 mm in adults/adolescents)
  - neurofibromas
- Look at the eyes:
  - Lisch nodules/iris hamartomas
  - optic glioma
- Look for a hearing aid
- Examine the back for scoliosis
  Offer to check the BP – can have phaeochromocytoma (tumour of adrenal medulla) or renal artery stenosis
- Look at relatives – does the mother have similar skin lesions?

Type 1

- > 6 café-au-lait spots
- Axillary freckling
- Nodular neurofibromata (after puberty)
- Other features include learning disabilities and epilepsy

Type 2

- Bilateral acoustic neuroma
- Deafness
- Cerebellopontine angle tumour

*From Lissauer T, Clayden G. Neurological disorders. In: *Illustrated Textbook of Paediatrics*, 2nd edn. London: Mosby, 2001, p. 379–80

- Associated features include hypertension due to renal artery stenosis and phaeochromocytoma, rarely sarcomatous change

*What do you know about the inheritance?**

Type 1 (gene found on chromosome 17) and type 2 (chromosome 22). Inheritance is autosomal dominant or it may arise from a spontaneous mutation. If there is a known mutation in the family, then antenatal testing can be offered.

What treatment is available?

Treatment is aimed at alleviating symptoms, particularly pressure symptoms of tumours on nerves, bone and in the brain. This may involve surgery. Occasionally tumours can become malignant and chemotherapy or radiotherapy may be needed. MRI scans can detect lesions such as acoustic neuromas when they are very small so that they can be removed early.

Further information and support can be found at: www.nfauk.org.

Cerebellar problems

- **Signs:**
  - start by talking to the child – you may notice dysarthria
  - check eye movements for nystagmus
- Next examine **gait:**
  - ataxic/trunk ataxia?
  - check for heel-to-toe walking
- **Impaired coordination:**
  - on finger–nose testing
  - intention tremor
  - past pointing
  - dysdiadochokinesis (testing the ability to perform rapidly alternating movements)
  - impaired coordination on heel–shin testing

Look for other clues:

- Bruising or other evidence of falls
- Signs of neurosurgical scars/shunts

*From Lissauer T, Clayden G. Neurocutaneous syndromes. In: *Illustrated Textbook of Paediatrics*, 2nd edn. London: Mosby, 2001, p. 381–2.

- Evidence of chemotherapy or radiotherapy
- Look at the feet – Friedreich's ataxia is associated with pes cavus
- State you would like to examine the vision and fundi – Friedreich's ataxia may be associated with optic atrophy

What is your differential diagnosis of cerebellar signs in a child?

- Neoplastic lesion/space-occupying lesion in cerebellum, e.g. neuroblastoma
- After infections, e.g. varicella causing a cerebellar encephalopathy
- Toxins, e.g. alcohol, phenytoin
- Ataxic cerebral palsy
- Spinocerebellar atrophy/Friedreich's ataxia
- Ataxia telangiectasia

What other associations are there with Friedreich's ataxia?

- Ataxia
- Loss of proprioception and vibration
- Loss of tendon reflexes
- Pes cavus
- Diabetes
- Optic atrophy
- Cardiomyopathy

Often presents between the age of 8 and 15 years.

What do you know of the inheritance of Friedreich's ataxia?

Autosomal recessive.

Hereditary sensory motor neuropathy (HSMN)

Also known as Charcot–Marie–Tooth/peroneal muscular atrophy.

Observation

- Callipers/foot splints/arch supports
- Gait – high stepping gait of foot drop
- Champagne bottle legs – distal/peroneal muscle wasting
- Pes cavus – claw toes

- Claw hands/wasting of small muscles of the hands
- Evidence of neuropathic ulcers on feet/burns on hands
- Inspection of back for scoliosis

Examination

- Palpable peripheral nerves in some patients
- Tone, power, reflexes, sensation:
  - muscle weakness
  - loss of knee and ankle reflexes
  - impaired proprioception/sensation

Other associated features

Occasionally associated with retinitis pigmentosa, optic atrophy or hearing problems.

What do you know about the inheritance?

Different forms, e.g. HSMN-1 and -2. Variable inheritance – autosomal dominant, autosomal recessive and X-linked forms.

How would you diagnose the condition?

- Nerve conduction studies
- Genetic testing

How would you manage a child with HSMN?

- Genetic counselling
- Physiotherapy
- Footwear/podiatry involvement, importance of looking after feet
- Corrective foot/scoliosis surgery may be required
- Follow-up by orthopaedics
- Calipers or walking aids may be required
- Consider a medic alert bracelet as in the event of an emergency, anaesthetists would need to know about the condition (www.medicalert.org.uk)
- Support groups/further information is available at, for example, www.cmt.org.uk

Further reading

Bellman M, Kennedy N (eds). *Paediatrics and Child Health: A Textbook for the DCH*. London: Churchill Livingstone, 2000: p. 87, 214.

Roach ES, DiMario FJ, Kandt RS, Northrup H. Tuberose Sclerosis Consensus Conference: Recommendations for diagnostic evaluation. *J Child Neurol* 1999;**14**:401–7.

Stephenson T, Wallace H, Thomson A. *Clinical Paediatrics for Postgraduate Examinations*, 3rd edn. Edinburgh: Churchill Livingstone, 2002: p. 242–3.

Anchor statement:

	Expected standard/ CLEAR PASS	PASS
PART A: RAPPORT	Full greeting and introduction Clarifies role and agrees aims and objectives Good eye contact and posture. Perceived to be actively listening (nod, etc.) with verbal and non-verbal cues Appropriate level of confidence, empathetic nature, putting parent/child at ease	Adequately performed but not fully fluent in conducting interview
PART A: EXAMINATION OF CHILD	Well structured and systematic approach Clear instructions given to child Accurate identification of normal development Good summary of findings and key priorities. Covers relevant aspects of case, including parent-held record, and delivers appropriate explanation	Reasonably systematic approach Identifies features of normal development Adequate though not complete summary of findings and key priorities Covers main relevant aspects of case and delivers adequate explanation
PART B: DISCUSSION OF PROBLEMS OF CHILD DEVELOPMENT	Evidence of knowledge in a clinical setting Suggests appropriate investigations and referral	Reasonable clinical thinking Appropriate investigations and referral

Child development

BARE FAIL	CLEAR FAIL	UNACCEPTABLE
Incomplete or hesitant greeting and introduction Inadequate identification of role, aims and objectives Poor eye contact and posture. Not perceived to be actively listening (nod, etc.) with verbal and non-verbal cues Does not show appropriate level of confidence, empathetic nature or putting parent/child at ease.	Significant components omitted or not achieved	Dismissive of parent/child concerns. Fails to put parent or child at ease
Hesitant examination covering main points but leaves out important tasks Incorrect conclusion	Poorly organized, inappropriate developmental examination Poor organization of child. Unable to recognize relevance of normal/abnormal signs Incorrect explanation	Completely unstructured assessment with slow hesitant approach. Failure to demonstrate to child Serious inadequacy in developmental skills or inability to interpret any findings
Some identification of further investigation, referral or treatment, but evidence of muddled thinking	Little clinical knowledge Poor identification of possible problems Lack of clarity of future planning	Serious deficiencies in knowledge and understanding of child development assessment

4 Developmental assessment

The DCH aims to test primary care paediatrics. Particularly important is the syllabus statement: *'Principles of health surveillance; normal physical, mental and emotional growth and development. Minor abnormalities and their management'* (www.rcpch.ac.uk/Examinations/DCH/DCH-Content-Syllabus--General-Info).

It can be difficult to perform a comprehensive developmental assessment in only 8 minutes, but using a systematic approach you should be able to make a good estimate of the child's age, or if this has been given to you, assess whether their development is normal. The examiners will offer direction if appropriate.

Remember, a child may have a global developmental delay or be delayed in a specific area, such as motor development. By getting down to the child's level and joining them in their play, you should be able gently to guide them to illustrate key milestones. *'Candidates should be able to set up an age appropriate situation around the child through which development can be observed with a minimum of intervention'* (www.rcpch.ac.uk/Examinations/DCH/DCH-Content-Syllabus--General-Info).

Break down your assessment into four main areas and ensure that you touch on all of these in your examination.

- Gross motor
- Fine motor and vision
- Hearing and communication
- Socialization

Also consider:

- Asking to see the red book (Personal Child Health Record – PCHR)

- Offering to measure weight, head circumference and height and plot these on a growth chart. (Be able to interpret and plot growth charts. Understand how to calculate mid-parental height and therefore the target centile range)

Be flexible in the order that you test developmental milestones. Do not allow the child to get bored. Keep introducing new toys or things to do. Praise and encourage the child at each step. Smile and make the tasks into a game where possible.

Although it is necessary to check that the examiner is happy for you to ask the mother/carer questions, it may be helpful to ask her a couple of questions whilst observing the child during your examination. However, where possible it is essential to demonstrate to the examiner the milestones attributed to the child by the parent or carer.

How to revise/prepare for this station

This chapter does not aim to provide comprehensive teaching about aspects of development but rather to provide an overview and basic framework for the exam. Most paediatric textbooks have detailed tables of milestones and ages. Find one that you like and learn the milestones. Familiarity with the milestones will make it easy for you to find things that a child can do, then something that they cannot and thereby to narrow down their likely age.

- Practise your developmental assessment on children as often as possible – sit in the play area of the ward or outpatients and play with children of different ages. They will happily show you what they can and cannot draw/demonstrate building towers, etc.
- Practise baby checks – neonate and 6 weeks
- Sit in developmental/community paediatric clinics
- Have an idea in your head of what children of different ages should be able to do: neonate, 6 weeks, 6 months, 8 months, 1 year, 2 years, 3 years, 4 years and 5 years
- Try and attend some audiology clinics
- The ophthalmology department may hold a paediatric clinic where you will observe lots of children with squints. Sitting in with the orthoptist will familiarize you with the cover test/assessing squints

There is no substitute for practice. It will be obvious to the examiners if you have not practised these skills.

Use a systematic approach

The examiners will be marking you on your rapport – which includes your introduction, your ability to act with confidence, your body language and empathy, as well as your communication skills.

They will also mark you on your general approach and whether it is systematic; whether you communicate clearly what you wish a child to do; and your ability to identify normal/abnormal development. They will then be looking for your ability to explain/summarize the findings and decide on a sensible management plan such as investigations or referral (www.rcpch.ac.uk/Examinations/DCH/DCH-Clinical-Structure).

Think about the approach you would take in the following station scenarios:

- 'Please examine this child – she is not walking at 18 months'
- 'This boy's parents are concerned about his vision – please assess him'
- 'Polly's teachers are concerned about her speech – please assess her'
- 'Please examine this baby – mum is concerned about his hearing'
- 'Please assess this baby/toddler/young child's development'

Even if the abnormality appears to be in one area only, you will need quickly to check other areas to ensure that the child does not have a global developmental delay. However, do listen carefully to the examiner's instructions. If doing a full developmental assessment on a young child, you may need to describe some aspects of it to the examiner; e.g. 'I have not noticed any problems with his hearing but I would like to ask mum about any concerns she has and perform a formal screening test such as the distraction test'. The examiner may reply, 'You do not need to perform that now but could you tell me the basic principles please.'

Do not be surprised to encounter both normal children and those with developmental delay in the exam. Be confident when presenting your findings.

6-week baby check

The basic outline of a 6-week baby check is listed below. The syllabus does mention, *'The care of the normal newborn. The early detection of abnormalities and their management'* (www.rcpch.ac.uk/Examinations/DCH/DCH-Content-Syllabus--General-Info).

Overall inspection – is the baby well and alert? Look for signs of jaundice, dehydration or any obvious physical abnormalities

- **Fontanelle** – check the anterior and posterior fontanelle (closed at term) and that they are not sunken (dehydration) or bulging (raised intracranial pressure)
- **Eyes** – red reflex, fixing and following, squint
- **Ears**– any obvious abnormalities
- **Facies** – symmetry, low set ears, epicanthic folds, protuberant tongue, hair line
- **Palate** – inspect, ask mum about feeding difficulties and feel gently with a clean finger
- **Chest** – auscultate/inspect
- **Arms and hands** – look for any obvious problems such as polydactyly, syndactyly, single palmar crease, incurving little finger
- **Abdomen** – palpation, distension, masses, hernia, scars
- **Umbilicus** – check clean and dry. Check for umbilical granuloma, umbilical hernia
- **Heart sounds** – check for any murmurs
- **Femoral pulses** – check both are equal
- **Hips** – Barlow's and Ortolani's tests check for dislocated or dislocatable/ clicky hips (Fig. 4.1)
- **Genitalia** – look for ambiguous genitalia (important as can be associated with congenital adrenal hyperplasia and a life-threatening salt-losing crisis), hypospadias (important to detect as parents should not have their child circumcised as may need foreskin for corrective surgery)
- **Testis** – check both are descended. If not then follow-up and if persistently undescended then will need to refer for surgery (which is usually carried out before 1 year old)
- **Anus** – patency, ask about passage of meconium. Delayed passage after birth for example may be associated with cystic fibrosis
- **Legs and feet** – look for equal leg length and symmetrical hip creases, talipes, femoral torsion, polydactyly. If the talipes is fixed, then refer. If positional, you can refer to a physiotherapist who can show the parents some stretching exercises
- **Sacrum** – look for any pits/moles which may indicate spina bifida
- **Skin** – note any birthmarks, e.g. strawberry naevus (Fig. 4.2) (usually regress and should be left alone unless obstructing vision or breathing/interfering with feeding), port wine stain (cavernous haemangioma) – usually do not fade and may need cosmetic laser treatment. If in trigeminal nerve distribution, may be associated with Sturge–Weber syndrome whereby there are associated intracranial abnormalities with epilepsy and intellectual impairment (Fig. 4.3) (see Chapter 2)
- **Spine** – run finger down spine, holding the baby in ventral suspension
- **Head control**

- **Stepping reflex** – hold baby upright and gently place feet on firm surface. Baby should lift feet in a stepping motion. Alternatively brush the baby's shins/dorsum of feet against the side of the couch and they should make a stepping motion
- **Grasp reflex** – stroke palm and they will grip your finger
- **Moro** – support the baby supine and with one hand under the head. Quickly lower the baby's head just a fraction and you will notice a flinging motion of both arms – startle reflex. This shows that both arms are moving symmetrically, and if not, may pick up lesions such as a brachial plexus injury sustained at birth
- **Head circumference and weight** (offer to plot in Personal Child Health Record – red book)

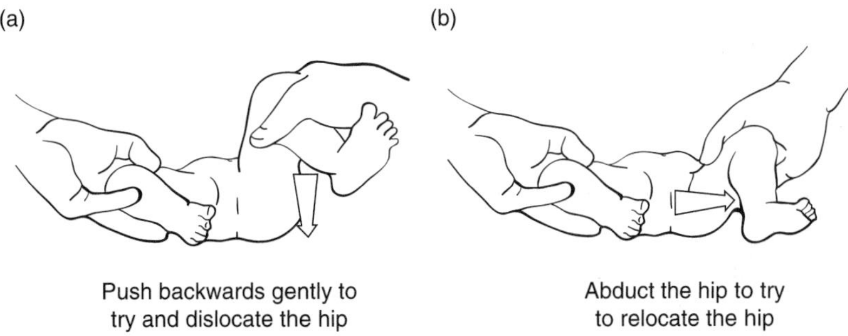
(a)
(b)
Push backwards gently to try and dislocate the hip
Abduct the hip to try to relocate the hip

FIGURE 4.1 (a) Barlow and (b) Ortolani tests.

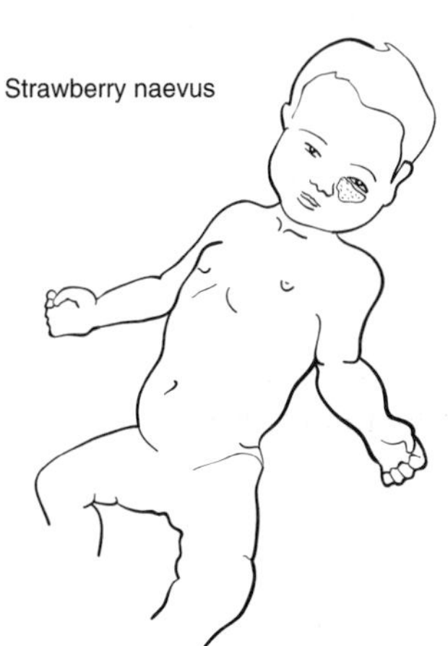
Strawberry naevus

FIGURE 4.2 Strawberry naevus. May present as a large pink lesion on the face as shown (or hidden behind the hairline or on the body).

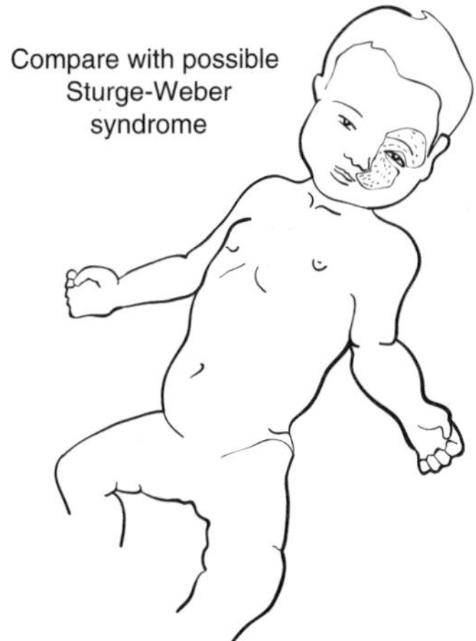
Compare with possible Sturge-Weber syndrome

FIGURE 4.3 Sturge-Weber lesion. Has a similar appearance to strawberry naevus, but is more extensive and occurs in the distribution of the trigeminal nerve.

Questions

- Ask about family history of hip problems, heart problems or hearing/vision problems, including squint
- Check that the child has received vitamin K (oral or IM, be able to discuss routes and timing of administration and the surrounding controversy)
- Discuss immunizations
- Check that no problems were picked up on antenatal scans
- Check that no problems were detected at neonatal hearing test
- Ask mother if she has any concerns
- Watch for signs of postnatal depression, e.g. Edinburgh Postnatal Depression Score (a calculator for this can be found on www.patient.co.uk)

Developmental assessment

Inspection

- Any dysmorphic facies?
- Squint?
- Hearing aid?
- Other clues such as hemiplegia

Gross motor assessment

- Pulling to sit – head lag
- Lifting baby prone with hand supporting underneath – holding head in line with body at 6 weeks
- Stepping reflex – hold baby upright under arms; when feet are brought into contact with hard surface, baby will make stepping movements
- Moro reflex
- Grasp reflex

How might a child with delayed motor development present?

A child with delayed motor development often presents as a floppy infant with head lag and who is unable to sit unsupported. The child may show early hand preference and scissoring of the legs when lifted.

They may not be walking at 18 months and may have had crawling variants such as bottom shuffling. *Note*: Not all bottom shufflers go on to have problems with their motor development. Bottom shufflers may, however, be late walkers (may not walk until 18–24 months). This may run in families. There may be

TABLE 4.1 Gross motor milestones

Milestone	Average age achieved
Pushing up on arms when prone	3 months
Reaching for objects – bringing them to midline	3 months (should not show hand preference)
Rolling – front to back and back to front	4–6 months
Sitting	6–8 months
Crawling	9 months (look for unusual variants such as bottom shuffling that may lead to later walking)
Pulling to stand	9 months
Cruising	12 months
Walking	15 months
Can stoop and pick up ball	18 months
Kicking/throw ball	18 months
Stairs	2 years
Ride a tricycle	3 years
Jumping/hopping	4 years

no other abnormalities but because of the link with cerebral palsy a careful examination should be carried out.

What may be the cause of developmental delay?

- Neurological problems such as cerebral palsy
- Spinal disorders such as spina bifida or spinal muscular atrophy
- Muscular disorders such as muscular dystrophy
- Myopathies such as myotonic dystrophy
- Chromosome disorders such as trisomy 21 which is associated with hypotonia
- Orthopaedic disorders such as dislocated hips or limb problems, e.g. arthrogryposis multiplex
- As part of a global developmental delay

Possible physical factors in global developmental delay

- Chromosome abnormality, e.g. trisomy 21
- Congenital infection
- Neonatal cerebral insult such as trauma, hypoxia, severe infection
- Use of drugs, alcohol, teratogenic medication in pregnancy
- Physical health and nutrition
- Metabolic defects
- Brain malformation

It is important that you understand the social determinants of developmental delay as well as those that are based on physical pathology (www.rcpch.ac.uk/Examinations/DCH/DCH-Content-Syllabus--General-Info).

Possible psychological/social factors in developmental delay

- Abuse
- Neglect
- Postnatal depression
- Large family/busy mother – child left sitting in chair/cot all day will not be able to explore surroundings/advance their motor skills, e.g. learning to walk
- A child who has no adult interaction may show language delay
- Cultural differences

Fine motor

- Palmar grasp – 4–6 months
- Pincer grip – scatter some hundreds and thousands or offer a small raisin – 9 months
- Bricks – ask the child to build a tower

TABLE 4.2 Drawing (fine motor) milestones

Milestone	Average age
Scribble	15 months
Line	2 years
Circle	3 years
Cross	3 years
Square	4 years
Person – stick figure	4 years
Triangle	5 years

TABLE 4.3 Tower building with bricks (fine motor) milestones

Milestone	Average age
3 bricks	18 months
6 bricks	2 years
9 bricks	3 years

Hearing

Testing hearing depends on age:

- At birth – neonatal testing is usually carried out by otoacoustic emission testing or brainstem evoked potentials
- Auditory brainstem response – measures EEG waves produced in response to clicks from an electrode on the baby's scalp
- Evoked otoacoustic emissions – uses a microphone to detect sound waves emitted from hair cells in the cochlea

The red book (Personal Child Health Record) contains screening questions for parents 'Can your child hear?'. Information can also be obtained from the NHS Newborn Hearing Screening Programme website (http://hearing.screening.nhs.uk/surveillance).

The DCH syllabus provides useful guidance on the knowledge expected for hearing and vision testing for the DCH (www.rcpch.ac.uk/Examinations/DCH/DCH-Content-Syllabus--General-Info).

Distraction testing – best at around 9 months (Fig. 4.4).

You may be asked to demonstrate the principles of this/describe it, but not to perform it in the exam. Try and watch it being done in the audiology clinic. For babies who are now screened at birth, this is no longer a routine test.

- Sound proof room
- One relative only
- No distractions
- Child sitting far forward on mother's knee
- Assistant distracts the child, e.g. by moving coloured balls in her hands
- Assistant is then still and quiet, and a noise such as from a rattle (e.g. a Manchester rattle) is made just out of the child's vision at a set distance from either the right or left ear (on metre)
- Watch for a reaction from the child (turning to look for the source of the noise)
- A meter will enable frequencies and volumes to be varied and recorded

McCormack toy testing – age range $2^1/_2$ – 4 years (speech discrimination)

Understand the principles and if possible go and observe in the audiology clinic.

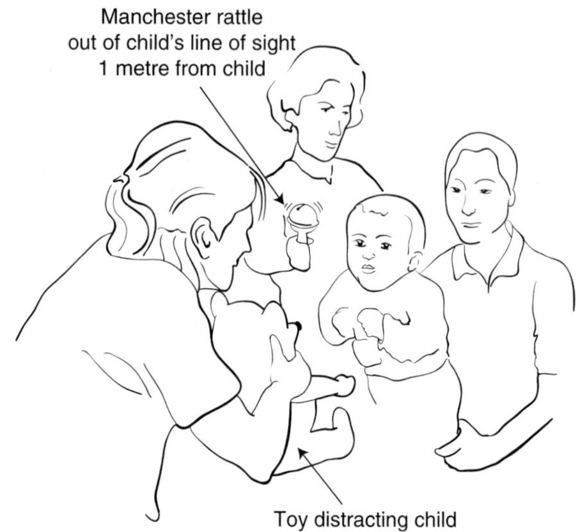

FIGURE 4.4 Distraction test. Nowadays rattle is often replaced by an electronic 'warbler'.

- There are specially made up sets of similar sounding words, e.g. horse/fork, key/tree
- First the examiner checks that the child knows what each object is
- Then, whilst covering their mouth so that the child cannot lip read, the examiner asks the child to identify various objects, e.g. 'show me the horse'
- Child then points to the correct object
- Examiner adjusts the volume of their voice and an assistant can use a decibel meter to record the volume
- Examiner should not use any visual clues, e.g. looking at the object they want the child to point to
- Children should get at least 8/10 correct

Younger children can perform a similar test with familiar objects, e.g. 'where is mummy?', 'where is teddy?', 'give the cup to teddy', after first checking their understanding of the object names (18–30 months).

Threshold audiometry (performance/conditioning test) – age range $2^1/_2 – 3^1/_2$ years

Listening for sounds of varying intensity/frequency – younger children can be encouraged to put bricks in a box or men in a boat when they hear a noise (either pure tone audiometry, warble or voice commands), turning the test into a game and keeping the child interested. The levels are checked with a sound meter.

Initially demonstrate the exercise to the child, then help the child to carry out the task, then gradually reduce assistance until there are no visual cues and the child is carrying out the exercise alone. The child should be praised every time they correctly perform the task.

Bone conduction can be compared to air conduction if a special headset is used.

Impedence testing

This uses a small piece of equipment that fits in the child's ear. Useful for glue ear (chronic secretory otitis media) which gives a flat curve.

Ensure that you can confidently perform an ear examination (Fig. 4.5).

Support and information for parents can be obtained from National Deaf Children's Society at www.ndcs.org.uk. Many aids can be provided to help a deaf child, including listening and alerting devices, subtitles, sign language

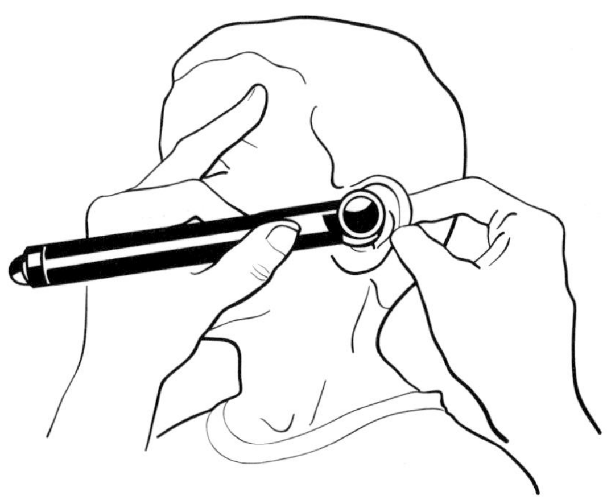

FIGURE 4.5 Examination of the ear with auroscope.

Risk factors for hearing loss

- Drugs, e.g. gentamicin used on SCBU
- Recurrent infections
- Otitis media with effusion
- Chronic secretory otitis media
- Congenital – infections, e.g. cytomegalovirus (CMV)
- Hereditary – positive family history, Down's syndrome
- Prematurity
- Congenital abnormalities of head and neck development
- Kernicterus
- Meningitis – especially pneumococcal
- Developmental delay

tuition, communication technology, radio aids, hearing dogs, hearing aids, cochlear implants and benefits.

Vision

Take parental concerns about visual impairment very seriously.

Note: severe visual impairment will impact on other aspects of development, and may be associated with underlying disorders such as Down's syndrome or cerebral palsy.

Visual loss may be hereditary and progressive, such as retinitis pigmentosa. Families may need to be referred for genetic counselling.

Be aware when testing vision that the room should be well illuminated. The child's age and reading ability will determine which tests can be used (see below). Think about distance, near and colour vision.

Inspection for signs of visual problems

- Obvious abnormalities surrounding the eye, e.g. large strawberry naevus, ptosis
- Iris abnormalities, e.g. coloboma (defect in iris)
- Manifest squint (obvious)
- Visual inattention
- Random eye movements
- Nystagmus
- Photophobia

- Loss of red reflex (leucocoria)
- Not smiling responsively

*Acuity assessment**

If the child is wearing glasses, test their acuity with them on to assess their corrected vision.

- From newborn – fixing and following, preference for patterned objects
- From 6 months – reaching well for toys
- From 9 months – picking up hundreds and thousands/pieces of fluff from the carpet
- From 2 years – matching picture cards. When testing the child who cannot yet read letters, pictures of reducing size can be shown from a distance and the child asked to point to a similar picture on a card in front of them
- From 3 years – can match letters using single letter charts (Sheridan and Gardner)
- From 5 years – can read a Snellen chart

Squints

- Look at the position of the light on both corneas – check for the light reflex (should fall in the same place in both eyes)
- **Cover test** – if there is a manifest/obvious squint, cover the eye that is fixing on the object. The deviated eye should move to take up fixation
- **Cover–uncover test**. If there is a latent squint, when you cover up one eye it stops focusing on the object and may drift out. When the eye is uncovered again, it will be seen to move back to take up fixation

There are two types of squint:

- **Concomitant** (non-paralytic) (Fig. 4.6):
  - convergent (esotropia)
  - divergent (exotropia)
  - alternating
- **Incomitant** (paralytic) – cranial nerve palsies

Pseudosquint due to prominent epicanthic folds is a fairly common finding in young babies, but if any doubt exists always refer to an orthoptist or ophthalmologist.

*From Lissauer T, Clayden G. Testing vision at different ages. In: *Illustrated Textbook of Paediatrics*, 2nd edn. London: Mosby, 2001, p. 35.

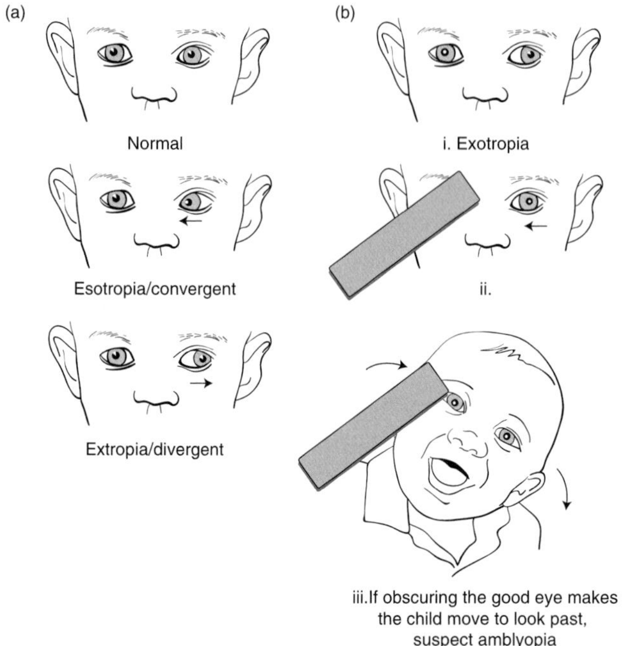

FIGURE 4.6 (a) Types of concomitant squint. (b) Cover test.

Colour vision assessment

Have a look at a set of Ishihara plates and learn how to interpret the results. The test consists of up to 36 cards. The patient is asked to read the hidden numbers on the cards. Eight or more errors indicate that there is a problem with colour vision.

Visual fields

In the older child, visual fields can be assessed with confrontation, as you would for an adult.

Loss of red reflex

This may be seen in family photographs. It requires urgent referral (see Fig. 4.7).

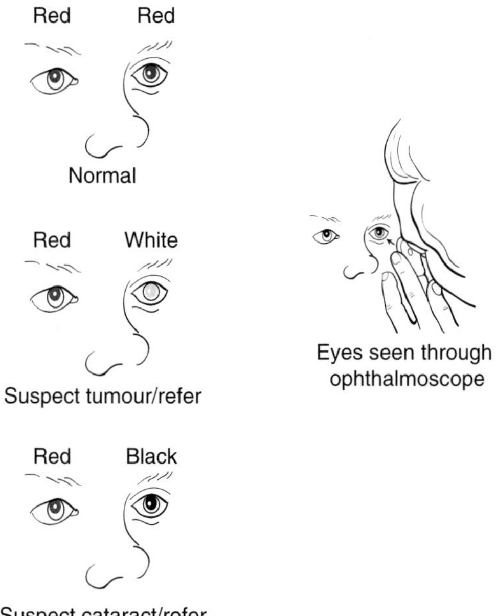

FIGURE 4.7 Red reflex abnormalities.

Causes of and risk factors for visual impairment

- **Causes:**
  - retinoblastoma
  - cataract
  - retinopathy of prematurity
  - inflammatory/infectious conditions
  - chromosome disorders
  - squint leading to amblyopia
  - amblyopia from obstructed vision, e.g. large strawberry naevus
- **Risk factors:**
  - prematurity
  - cerebral palsy
  - chromosome disorders such as Down's syndrome
  - genetic/family history
  - congenital infection

Support and information for parents can be obtained from the National Blind Children's Society at www.nbcs.org.uk.

Speech

'Candidates should be able through history taking and/or observation to give an account of the child's language development' (www.rcpch.ac.uk/Examinations/DCH/DCH-Content-Syllabus--General-Info).

Listen to the child's speech.

TABLE 4.4 Language milestones

Milestone	Average age
Consonant babble – baba, dada,	6 months
Using words with meaning, e.g. mama	9 months
Few words	12 months
50 words	18 months
Phrases	2 years
Sentences	3 years
Ask if they know their name?	3 years
Recognizes colours?	3 years
Names colours?	4 years
Can count?	4 years

If the child is older, perhaps pick up a picture book and ask them to point to things (comprehension), ask them what the objects in the picture are and ask them to describe what is happening in the story. Children older than 2 years should be able to tell simple stories from pictures.

Comment on their understanding (comprehension), expression (e.g. single words/joined words/sentences) and articulation.

Common problems that may need referral to a speech therapist include specific problems with articulation, stammers and speech delay. Remember to look for an *underlying* cause:

- Hearing loss
- Social factors, e.g. bullying/abuse/neglect
- Physical reason – head and neck abnormalities, cleft lip or palate, macroglossia
- Global delay

Socialization

You may be able to observe some behaviour but also ask the examiner if you may ask the mother a few questions.

TABLE 4.5 Socialization milestones

Milestone	Average age
Smile	6 weeks
Wave bye-bye	9 months
Indicates wants	9 months
Clap hands	9 months
Hold cup	12 months
Feed themselves with fingers, e.g. rusk	6 months
Use spoon	15 months
Continence – dry by day	2 years
Dry by day and night	3 years
Dresses with help	3 years

Play – symbolic? Are there any toys in the room you could watch the child playing with? E.g. pretending to cook/feed teddy some food/ brush the doll's hair. If not, ask the mother about the child's play.

Know the age limits and key referral criteria

TABLE 4.6 Age limits for key developmental milestones

Not sitting alone	9 months
Not standing	12 months
Not walking	18 months (some variants of crawling may be associated with later walking)
Not reaching	5–6 months
No pincer grip	10–12 months
Not babbling	7 months
Not 6 words	18 months
Not smiling	8 weeks

Note: in very premature babies you may need to allow for their prematurity in the timing of their milestones.

Know the common schedules of child health surveillance

As well as being familiar with the basic newborn and 6-week checks, be aware of other screening tests that are carried out, such as neonatal hearing testing, the 5-day heel–prick test and measurement of weight and head circumference by health visitors. GPs no longer carry out formal developmental checks after the 6-week check.

Familiarize yourself with the red book (Personal Child Health Record). This keeps a record of developmental checks, weights, head circumferences and provides parents with information and advice. It can give you useful information about the types of questions that are used to flag up problems, e.g. 'Can your baby see?' or 'Can your baby hear?'

Know what investigations may be needed?

- MRI scan
- EEG
- Metabolic screen, e.g. for inherited disorders of metabolism; usually requires testing of blood and urine samples
- Chromosomes, e.g. looking for trisomy 21, fragile X syndrome
- Thyroid function tests – hypothyroidism
- Creatine kinase – to screen for Duchenne's muscular dystrophy
- EMG
- Nerve conduction studies – hereditary sensory motor neuropathy (Charcot–Marie–Tooth)

Know the services available in your area to help children identified with motor, sensory, educational and emotional disability

These may include:

- Community/hospital paediatricians/paediatric surgeons
- Health visitors
- Specialist nurses
- Paediatric audiologists/ENT
- Paediatric orthoptists/ophthalmology
- Social workers
- Educational psychologists
- Statementing – special schools or support
- Physiotherapists
- Occupational therapists

- Speech and language therapists
- Dietician
- Support groups
- Respite care
- Financial support – allowances
- Specific services and education/support/equipment for those with visual or auditory problems

Further reading

Beattie M, Clark A, Smith A. Child development. In: *Short Cases for the Paediatric Membership*. Knutsford: PasTest, 1999.

Cox JL, Holden J, Sagovsky R. Development of the 10-item Edinburgh Postnatal Depression Scale. *Br J Psychiatry* 1987;**150**:782–6.

Lissauer T, Clayden G. Child development, hearing and vision. In: *Illustrated Textbook of Paediatrics*, 2nd edn. Edinburgh: Churchill Livingstone, 2001.

Murray L, Carothers A. The validation of the Edinburgh Post-natal Depression Scale on a community sample. *Br J Psychiatry* 1990;**157**:288–90.

Anchor statement:

	Expected standard/ CLEAR PASS	PASS
PART A: RAPPORT	Full greeting and introduction Clarifies role and agrees aims and objectives Good eye contact and posture Perceived to be actively listening (nod, etc.) with verbal and non-verbal cues Appropriate level of confidence Empathetic nature. Putting parent/child at ease	Adequately performed but not fully fluent in conducting interview
PART A: FOCUSED HISTORY	Asks clear questions pertinent to the case Open and closed questions. Parent, child and examiner can hear and understand fully Appropriate answers to parents' questions Structured questions, avoids jargon, picks up verbal and non-verbal cues Succinct summary of key issues	Questions reasonable and cover essential issues but omits occasional essential points Overall approach structured Appropriate style of questioning Main points summarized
PART B: SUMMARY, MANAGEMENT PLANNING AND CLOSURE	Invites further questions Summarizes Gives accurate information Explores options for management Provides appropriate further contact information Refers to other agencies	Summarizes most of the important points and suggests **best** management strategy Provides some information about other services and future plan Deals with uncertainty in diagnosis or management

Focused history

BARE FAIL	CLEAR FAIL	UNACCEPTABLE
Incomplete or hesitant greeting and introduction Inadequate identification of role, aims and objectives Poor eye contact and posture. Not perceived to be actively listening (nod, etc.) with verbal and non-verbal cues Does not show appropriate level of confidence, empathetic nature or putting parent/child at ease	Significant components omitted or not achieved	Dismissive of parent/child concerns Fails to put parent or child at ease
Misses relevant information, which would make a difference to management if known Excessive use of closed questions Occasional use of jargon Summary incomplete	Asks irrelevant questions, poorly understood by parent and child Excessive use of jargon Does not seek the view of parent/child Very poor summary	Questions totally unrelated to the problem presented Shows no regard to the child/parent No summary
Incomplete summary of problems and inadequately planned management Does not relate management to child's/parents' needs or concerns Inadequate attempt to determine child/parent understanding	Poor summary Patient unsure of future plans Poor discussion of management options Poor exploration of parents' or child's views or desires about treatment Poor use of referral to other agencies	Abrupt ending Inaccurate information given Lack of regard for safe, ethical and effective treatments Poor arrangements for future contact

5 Focused history and management planning

This is a 13 minute station that aims to test your ability to take a focused history and discuss the management of a patient. You should be able to identify the main issues and concerns of the parent and child. After 8 minutes with the parent and child you will have 5 minutes with the examiner to summarize the case and discuss the management.

Examiners will be marking you on your rapport. Marks may be given for (www.rcpch.ac.uk/Examinations/DCH/DCH-Clinical-Structure):

- A full greeting and introduction
- Clarifying role and agreeing aims and objectives
- Good eye contact and posture
- Active listening, picking up on verbal and non-verbal cues
- Appropriate level of confidence
- Empathetic nature
- Putting parent/child at ease

If there is a child at the station, then fully involve them in the history taking, aiming for a relaxed discussion with *both* the child and the parent.

You will need to obtain a thorough history about the current problem as well as some background history. The station is not a test of your ability to take a complete history and you are unlikely to be asked to present everything that you have just learned to the examiner. If the parent or child asks a question during the history, then answer them.

Marks may be given for:

- Asking clear questions pertinent to the case
- Open and closed questions that the parent, child and examiner can hear and understand fully

- Appropriate answers to a parent's questions
- Structured questions, avoiding jargon, picking up verbal and non-verbal cues
- Succinct summary of key issues
- Inviting further questions
- Summarizing
- Giving accurate information
- Exploring options for management
- Providing further contact information
- Referral to other agencies

You should be familiar with the management of common childhood illnesses and chronic conditions (these stations often concern children with a chronic illness). This chapter gives examples of scenarios that you could practise with a colleague. Remember that this is a clinical examination and practise is vital. The scenarios also illustrate your need to think of the child and their family as a whole when planning the management. You should include psychological aspects, the need to refer to other agencies and the availability of other sources of information for the family, as well as the medical management.

Examples of history taking/management planning

Asthma history

Scenario 1

A couple and their 10-year-old son with asthma have just moved to your area. Please take a history so that you can plan his care.

Introduce yourself and establish a **rapport**. If the son is with his parents, interact with him too. Find out what he likes to be called.
Explain that you need to ask them some questions about his asthma so that you can ensure that he is properly managed.

Start with open-ended questions:
- How are things going with his asthma at the moment?
- Do they have any concerns?

Move on to more focused questions:
Determining the severity/history of his asthma
- How long has he had asthma?

- How bad is it – has hospital admission ever been necessary? Admission to intensive care unit?
- Courses of steroids?
- Time off school?
- Cough/disturbed sleep?
- Is he coping with physical education at school/keeping up with peers/friends when playing?
- Peak flow diary?
- Is he growing OK?

Current management
- What medication does he currently use?
- Is he happy with his spacer/inhaler type?
- How does he use it – washing out mouth after inhaled steroid use?

What tends to trigger his asthma?
- Hayfever?
- Allergies?
- Eczema?
- Pets?
- Smoking – parents? Smoky rooms?

Quick background history (depending on time available and what you feel is relevant)
- Past medical history (PMH)
- Meds
- Allergies
- Family history (FH) of asthma?
- Social history (SH) – family structure
- Immunizations
- Development/school
- Birth

Plan for care
- Who is he under? (practice asthma nurse/hospital paediatric respiratory clinic?)
- How often is he seen?
- Do they have a plan for what to do when he gets a cough/cold?

Summarize what you have discussed with them.
Ask if there are any more **questions?**

Depending on the answers you get it may be appropriate to:

- Arrange follow-up with asthma nurse/yourself
- Refer to paediatrician
- Ask them to keep a peak flow diary
- Review or alter medication
- Check inhaler techniques/teach about spacer
- Allergen/smoking advice
- Educate them so that they know what to do in an exacerbation (with written information)
- Offer information, e.g. websites/support groups

A useful website with leaflets and advice for children and parents is available at www.asthma.org.uk.

Familiarize yourself with the asthma guidelines – particularly helpful are the BTS/SIGN guidelines (www.brit-thoracic.org.uk, www.sign.ac.uk). The paediatric BNF has useful information on asthma medications and the stepwise approach that should be adopted (bnfc.org/bnfc).

Cystic fibrosis history

Refresh your knowledge before the exam by reading about the clinical features and management of cystic fibrosis in a paediatric textbook. Children with this condition are commonly encountered in the DCH and you should be able to examine and discuss in some detail the relevant clinical signs.

Scenario 2

Cheryl is a 13-year-old girl who is missing a lot of school due to her cystic fibrosis and she is losing weight. Mum is concerned. Please take a history of her condition and care so far, so that you can plan further management.

Introduce yourself to Cheryl and her mum and **explain** your role. Establish **rapport**.

Start with open-ended questions:

- What are mum's concerns?
- How does Cheryl see the problem?
- How much school does she miss? – Why? Is she falling behind? What would help her miss less school?
- Why do they think she is losing weight?

Move on to more focused questions:

- When was she diagnosed?
- How does it affect her now?
- What is her current management?
- Who is she under? (community specialist nurse, specialist centre, local paediatric team, community paediatrician, other specialists, e.g. gastroenterology)
- How often is she followed up?

In order to determine why she might be losing weight/missing school it may be helpful to consider one system at a time.

Respiratory

- Is she often off school with chest infections?
- Does she use inhalers? Antibiotics? Does she have a permanent line (e.g. portacath) for intravenous antibiotics?
- What physiotherapy does she do? Postural drainage? Does she do any at school?
- How many hospital admissions has she had?

Gastroenterology

- What dietary supplements does she take?
- How much weight has she lost?
- Does she take her Creon? (pancreatic enzyme supplement)
- How is her appetite?
- Opening bowels OK? Stool – any steatorrhoea? Rectal prolapse?
- Any abdominal pain or jaundice?

Cardiac

- Is she under a cardiologist?
- Has she had an echocardiogram?
- What is her exercise tolerance like?

Endocrine

- Any symptoms of diabetes?
- Has she been checked for diabetes?
- Where is she in relation to puberty?
- Has she had her adolescent growth spurt?

Psychological

- How is she coping with cystic fibrosis as a teenager?
- Any support groups in the area?
- Has she ever had any counselling?
- Does anything worry her or make her feel down?

- Does she suffer from low mood or tearfulness?
- Does she get embarrassed taking medications/doing physiotherapy at school?

You could then **summarize** the key points of the case and discuss the management of her cystic fibrosis.
Ask if she or her mother have any **questions.**

Depending on the answers you get it may be appropriate to:
- Discuss the need for further investigations into her weight loss
- Refer her to a hospital paediatrician and a dietician
- Increase her psychological well-being – counselling/support groups
- Liaise with community child health teams/school – to try and address school absence (explore possibility of home-based teaching when unwell)

She may be interested in looking at the Cystic Fibrosis Trust website which provides useful information/support (www.cftrust.org.uk).

Epilepsy history

Read about the common types of epilepsy in young children. Remember that children who have had a single fit are not usually diagnosed immediately with epilepsy or started on medications. For information on febrile convulsions, see Chapter 7.

Scenario 3

Sam is a 10-year-old with epilepsy. His mum is concerned about him going on a school trip as his epilepsy is not well controlled at present. Please take a history of his condition in order to plan his management.

Introduce yourself to Sam and his mum and build a **rapport.**
Explain that you understand her worries and that you will need to ask a few questions about her son's epilepsy in order to plan what to do about the school trip.

Start with open-ended questions:
- What will the trip involve?
- How will the children be supervised?
- Are the school trained in what to do if he fits? Do they carry rectal diazepam or buccal midazolam?

Move on to more focused questions:
- When was he diagnosed?

- What medication is he on?
- Any side effects?
- Compliance?
- Any recent change in medication?
- Follow-up/who under?
- Does he have an alert bracelet?
- Fit frequency?
- Triggers?
- Aura and warning signs?
- How do they treat fits?
- General development and progress at school
- Psychological effects – how he feels about the epilepsy?
- Any support? Ever been on outings with an epilepsy support group?
- How do his friends react?

Summarize what mum has told you and what her concerns are.
Ask if she has any more **questions?**

Depending on the answers you get it may be appropriate to discuss:

- Referral to a paediatrician for optimization of his medications
- Mum to check the level of supervision on the trip – negotiation about which activities would and would not be safe (e.g. lone swimming or cycling)
- Importance of compliance with medications
- Awareness by Sam of triggers, e.g. hunger/overtiredness
- Wearing a Medicalert bracelet
- Liaison with school (is there a school nurse?) and education for his school regarding management of his epilepsy
- Provision of emergency rectal diazepam/buccal midazolam
- Referral to epilepsy support groups

The website www.epilepsy.org.uk has lots of information for children, adolescents and their families, and for friends who may want to learn more.

Look at the BNF to familiarize yourself with the common antiepileptic drugs and their side effects (bnfc.org/bnfc), e.g.

- **Phenytoin** – gum hypertrophy, coarse facies, acne and hirsutism, tremor and ataxia
- **Carbamazepine** – blood disorders, drowsiness, visual disturbance
- **Sodium valproate** – liver toxicity, weight gain, nausea

Remember to educate teenage girls on contraception (enzyme induction makes hormonal contraception less effective and antiepileptic drugs can be teratogenic).

Diabetes history

> **Scenario 4**
>
> Brian has just moved to your area. He is a diabetic and is 14 years old. His dad has brought him in as he is concerned that his sugars are not well controlled and Brian is not really bothering to check his levels. Please take a focused history so that you can plan his care.

Introduce yourself to Brian and his dad and establish a **rapport**.
Explain that you would like to find out a bit more about his diabetes so that you can address their concerns.

Start with open-ended questions:
- What are dad's concerns about the diabetes at the moment?
- How does Brian feel about his diabetic control at the moment?

Move on to more focused questions:
- What treatment is he on at the moment?
- Does he give his own injections?
- Does he vary the sites of injections? Any problems with injection sites?
- When does he check his blood sugars? How does he feel about that?
- What sort of readings is he getting? Does he keep a diary?
- Does he ever check his urine for ketones?
- Does he ever miss doses?
- Any hypoglycaemic attacks (hypos)? What does he do if he gets a hypo? What warning does he get? Do family and school know how to treat one? Does he carry a source of sugar with him, e.g. Hypostop/Lucozade tablets?
- Has he ever been admitted with diabetic ketoacidosis?
- Does he know what to do if he is ill?
- What is his exercise level like/is he involved in any particular sport?
- Diet?
- Weight?
- Where is he in relation to puberty? Growth spurt?
- How does he manage his diabetes at school?
- How do his friends react?
- Does it bother him injecting at school?
- Psychological state?
- Any known problems with: injection sites?, feet?, eyes?, kidneys?

Ask Brian if he has any concerns/worries?

Summarize the main issues and concerns that have been raised.
Ask if there are any more **questions.**

Depending on the answers you get it may be appropriate to:
- Refer to a paediatrician
- Arrange follow-up with specialist diabetic nurse/yourself
- Consider testing thyroid function and performing a coeliac screen (increased incidence)
- Adjust medications/monitoring so they fit better into teenager's life
- Work on education about hypos/what to do when unwell
- Liaise with school – education on diabetes/management of hypos
- Refer to dietician
- Consider psychological support/referral to support group
- Offer advice on where to find more information on the Internet

The website www.diabetes.org.uk includes a section 'My life' which is geared to young people with diabetes; www.nice.org.uk has a quick reference guide titled 'Type 1 diabetes in children and young people,' and www.library.nhs.uk/diabetes has a very useful document called 'Approaching the parents of a child with diabetes.' The latter makes many suggestions for parents looking after a child with diabetes, e.g. they advise that rewards should be offered for sticking to the correct diet and complying with treatment. They should never depend on outcomes, e.g. HbA1C.

Enuresis history

Scenario 5

Donald's mum has come to see you about him as he is 7 years old and is still wetting the bed. Please take a history and plan further management.

Introduce yourself and establish a **rapport**.
Explain that you will need to ask some questions about Donald and then you will be able to decide how best to help him.

Start with open-ended questions:
- Ask about the problem and her concerns
- Why is she concerned now?
- What does she think is causing it?

Move on to more focused questions:

- History of potty training
- Is he dry during the day?
- Has he ever been dry at night?
- How often does he wet the bed?
- What do they do when he wets the bed? What have they tried? E.g. fluid restriction in the evening, waking to go to the loo when parents go to bed
- Is anything bothering him? Stress at school or home?
- Any symptoms of infection – tummy pains, fever or complaints of discomfort on passing urine?
- Any symptoms of diabetes? Increased fluid intake, thirst, weight change, infections?
- Problems with constipation?

Quick background history (depending on time available and what you feel is relevant)

- PMH – spina bifida, diabetes?
- Medications/allergies
- FH of enuresis? Brothers/sisters/father?
- SH – family structure? New baby? Any stress at home?
- Immunizations
- Development/school – any stress or concerns about school?
- Birth

Summarize the issues/concerns raised by mum.
Ask if there are any more **questions.**

Depending on the answers you get it may be appropriate to:

- Arrange to see Donald to perform an examination
- Talk to Donald about the problem/offer reassurance
- Perform further investigations including testing for diabetes and urinary infection
- Refer to specialist
- Offer psychological support
- Teach family behavioural techniques such as star charts
- Talk about fluids, e.g. drinking a reasonable amount in the day, avoiding fizzy drinks and using the toilet before bed
- Offer more specialized equipment such as pad alarms (usually only effective in 7 years+), waterproof sheeting

Discuss short-term medications such as desmopressin for school trips, etc. However, drugs are used less and less frequently. Tricyclics such as imipramine are now contraindicated due to the risk of serious cardiac arrhythmias in overdose and there has been a drug safety alert for desmopressin following its link to concerns about water retention and seizures (www.mhra.gov.uk; see below).

Inform them of websites/help groups and sources of further information/ leaflets, e.g. from ERIC ('Education and Resources for Improving Childhood incontinence') www.eric.org.uk.

Common treatment options for nocturnal enuresis

- **Dry bed training** refers to regimens that include enuresis alarms, waking routines, positive practice, cleanliness training, bladder training and rewards in various combinations
- **Star charts** are used as a record and incentive scheme, alone or with other treatments
- **Enuresis alarms,** which wake the child in the night at the onset of wetting, are a form of conditioning that may require several months of continual use to be effective
- **Desmopressin** is a synthetic analogue of antidiuretic hormone that reduces nocturnal urine output. It has a rapid onset making it suitable for short term use. It can be used alone or with an enuresis alarm. The indication has been withdrawn for the nasal spray form, Desmospray, due to the risk of side effects in overdose

Headache history

Scenario 6

Eleanor is missing a lot of school due to headaches. Her mother is concerned. Please take a history.

Introduce yourself to Eleanor and her mum and build a **rapport.**

Start with some open-ended questions:

- Tell me about the headaches
- What do they think is causing them?
- What are they worried about?
- How much school is she missing?
- Is she falling behind?

Move on to more focused questions:

- How long have the headaches been going on for? When did they first start?

- Any warning/triggers?
- Onset?
- Location?
- Character?
- How long do they last for?
- Any pattern to headaches? (Time of day/day of week? Worse first thing in the morning, better at weekends?)
- Any worse? Pattern changing?
- How does she look when she has the headache?
- Associated symptoms: vomiting, nausea, fever, photophobia, weight loss?
- How do they treat them? What helps? What makes them worse?

Any other problems or symptoms?
- Growing well/progress at school OK?
- Eyesight OK?
- Clumsiness, reading/writing deterioration?
- Enjoying school/recent change in school?
- Anything she does not like at school?
- Any bullying?

Quick background history (depending on time available and what you feel is relevant)
- PMH – any other illnesses
- Medications/allergies – overuse of analgesics? (analgesic or rebound headache)
- FH of migraines?
- SH – family structure? Any stress at home? Depression? Bereavement?
- Immunizations
- Development/school – any stress or concerns about school
- Birth

Summarize the issues/concerns raised by mum.
Ask if there are any more **questions.**

Depending on the answers you get it may be appropriate to:
- Arrange to examine Eleanor (check blood pressure, growth, neurological examination including fundi, dermatological exam for neurocutaneous lesions)
- Arrange an eye test
- Ask them to keep a diary of her symptoms
- Offer reassurance
- Explain that a scan is not necessary (unless there are red flags such as an abnormal neurological examination, seizures, a recent onset of severe

headache, early morning headaches, vomiting, deterioration in writing/school performance)
- Talk about migraines running in the family
- Talk about treatment
- Refer to paediatrician
- Liaise with the school
- Explore psychological issues
- Offer leaflets/sources of more information
- Offer a follow-up appointment

The UCL Institute of Child Health has produced some useful paediatric guidelines including one on 'headache' (www.ich.ucl.ac.uk).

Crying baby history

> **Scenario 7**
>
> Mrs Smith is concerned that her 2-month-old baby has been crying a lot over the last few weeks and she doesn't know what is wrong. Please take a history and explore her concerns.

Introduce yourself to Mum and build a **rapport.**

Start with some open-ended questions:
- Tell me about your new baby
- What does she think is causing the crying?
- What is she worried about?
- What does her health visitor/family think?

Move on to more focused questions:
- When does the crying occur?
- Time of day/night?
- Relationship to feeds?
- Are there periods of contentment?
- What does the baby look like – flushed/pale/draws legs up?
- What does she do when the baby cries?
- What seems to help?
- Feeding pattern – breast/bottle?
- How much milk? When?
- Is the baby gaining weight? Head circumference OK?
- Has she brought the Parent Held Child Health Record (red book) with her?

- What are the stools like?
- Wet nappies?
- Any vomiting?
- Any nappy rash or skin rashes?
- Any fever?
- Any other symptoms?

Quick background history (depending on time available and what you feel is relevant)
- Medications/allergies – what has she tried giving?
- FH – any other children? Similar problems when they were young?
- SH – family structure? Any stress at home? Any other children at home? Family support? Parents? Is husband/partner at home?

Birth history
- Any problems in neonatal period?
- Passed meconium in first 24 hours?
- Did the baby spend time in the special care baby unit?
- Was the baby born prematurely?

Psychological assessment
- Signs of postnatal depression?
- Is she coping with the tiredness?
- Does she get any help at night?
- Is the stress affecting her relationship with her husband/partner?
- What support does she have?

Summarize problem and mum's concerns.
Ask if there are any more **questions.**

Depending on the answers you get it may be appropriate to:
- Arrange to examine the baby to look for causes, e.g. nappy rash, oral thrush
- Check head circumference/weight and plot in Parent Held Child Health Record (red book)
- Arrange further investigations
- Refer to paediatrician
- Offer reassurance if this is a well baby who has periods of contentment and is gaining weight well
- Discuss remedies such as Infacol (simeticone) if the pattern of crying is mostly in the evenings and suggestive of colic – some mothers find it helps
- Is the baby overfed, prematurely weaned or inadvertently swallowing air at the end of a bottle feed? Advice on feeding may be needed
- Involve health visitor

- Arrange support for mum – encourage parents to get as much rest as possible, perhaps asking a family member to baby sit for a period
- Screen mum for postnatal depression
- Parenting groups for support
- Offer follow-up
- Offer sources of further information, e.g. Internet

Birth to Five (www.dh.gov.uk) is a very useful source of sensible advice on feeding, immunizations, childhood illnesses, child safety, child development, practical support and benefits for parents. The DCH covers common childhood problems and this source explains things in simple language which can help you explain various issues to parents in the communication as well as history stations. You could also suggest the book to a parent who wanted more information.

Scenarios to practise with a friend

Note: there is an overlap between topics that can appear in these stations and those that test communications skills.

- Child with a disability moving to your area
- Child with trisomy 21 (Down's)
- Poor eating/picky eater/obesity
- Behavioural problems such as tantrums, not sleeping, hyperactivity, autistic spectrum disorder
- Chronic abdominal pain
- Review of eczema
- Constipation
- Failure to thrive

Further reading

Diabetes Education Study Group *DESG. Teaching Letter No. 31*. Approaching the parents of a Child with Diabetes Mellitus. Diabetes Education Study Group (DESG) of the European Association for the Study of Diabetes (EASD). www.library.nhs.uk/diabetes.

British Thoracic Society and Scottish Intercollegiate Guidelines Network. *British Guideline on the Management of Asthma – A National Clinical Guideline*. Edinburgh: Scottish Intercollegiate Guidelines Network, 2008. www.sign.ac.uk/pdf/sign101.pdf.

Department of Health. *Birth to Five*. London: DH, 2007. www.dh.gov.uk.

Evan JHC. Evidence based management of nocturnal enuresis. *BMJ* 2001;**323**: 1167–9.

Gatrad AR, Sheikh A. Evidence based paediatrics: 10-minute consultation. Persistent crying in babies. *BMJ* 2004;**328**:330.

UCL Institute of Child Health. Headache Clinical Guideline. London: UCL Institute of Child Health, 2006. www.ich.ucl.ac.uk.

Khot A, Polmear A. Recurrent physical symptoms. In: *Practical General Practice*, 5th edn. London: Butterworth Heinemann, 2006: p. 77 (Excessive crying), 93 (Recurrent physical symptoms).

Lissauer T, Clayden G. *Illustrated Textbook of Paediatrics*, 2nd edn. London: Mosby, 2001, p. 228 (Respiratory disorders – patient education); 366–71 (Neurological disorders).

Meadow R, Newell S. *OSCE station: History taking – pain; Emotional and behavioural problems*. In: *Lecture Notes on Paediatrics*, 7th edn. Oxford: Blackwell Science, 2002.

National Institute for Health and Clinical Excellence. *Type 1 diabetes: diagnosis and management of type 1 diabetes in children, young people and adults. NICE clinical guidelines 15*. London: NICE, 2004.

van Dorp F, Simon C. Funny turns in small children. *InnovAiT* 2008;**1**:73–8.

Anchor statement: Structured oral

	Expected standard/ CLEAR PASS	PASS	BARE FAIL
DISCUSSION	Knowledge and its application in clinical setting Considers ethical issues Clear, appropriate and professional	Able to solve problems Reasonable clinical thinking	Some ability in problem solving Muddled clinical thinking

	FAIL	UNACCEPTABLE
DISCUSSION	Little ability in problem solving Muddled clinical thinking Examiner has to work hard to give assistance	Poor grasp of clinical concepts Argumentative or dogmatic in approach

6 The structured oral examination

This station tests the candidate's knowledge and attitudes concerning: '*Two topics: common paediatric problems, management, ethical [topics] and/or consent*' (www.rcpch.ac.uk/Examinations/DCH/DCH-Clinical-Structure) The station lasts 13 minutes and there are likely to be two examiners taking it in turns to mark and assess.

In this chapter we examine 10 likely topics not covered elsewhere in the book. These may be used as a framework for studying other topics which are relevant to primary care.

An excellent way to practise/revise for these stations is group discussion and/or timed mock oral examinations with seniors. The paediatric sections of either *The Oxford Handbook of General Practice* (2nd edn) or *The Oxford Handbook of Clinical Specialties* (7th edn) are useful sources of condensed information. However, it is a good idea to keep abreast of relevant NICE guidelines, such as those for fever in children, urinary infections and head injury.

During your paediatric job try to spend some time in community paediatrics. Here you may come across school nurses and their roles, the legal issues and medical examinations associated with adoption and fostering, child protection issues and 'statementing'. Attend the child protection training run by your trust. Consider how this would apply to you if working as a GP in the community, and how you would access child health surveillance and child protection services.

Child protection

What constitutes child abuse?

Four categories of child abuse are recognized and these often coexist:

- Physical abuse or non-accidental injury(NAI)
- Emotional abuse
- Sexual abuse
- Neglect

A fifth category is functional or induced illness in a child instigated by a parent or guardian. The term 'Munchausen's by proxy' for this has largely fallen out of favour.

How does the law protect children from abuse and neglect?

The Children Act 1989/2004:

- **Section 47**: provides for children at risk of significant harm (parents may be overruled)
- **Section 17**: provides for children in need of assistance to flourish (requires parental consent)

The Sexual Offences Act 2003 clarifies what is a sexual offence against a child, especially what may be classed as rape, and the Forced Marriages Act 2007 protects against forced marriages.

The Education Act 1981 provides legal guidance on education provision standards.

If you are worried that a child is at significant risk of harm, what can you do as a GP?

- Clearly communicate your concerns with appropriate members of your healthcare team, and document them clearly
- Call the appropriate child protection worker
- Be familiar with your local guidelines and your duties as a healthcare worker (www.everychildmatters.gov.uk), e.g. hospital admission may protect a child and allow a full assessment. Social services and the child protection team have a 24-hour on-call phone number
- If admission is refused, either by the parent/carer or by the admitting paediatrician, for any reason, social services can instigate a place of safety order, or the police can remove a child into police protection

What if you are not sure that there is a risk?

- Check with social services whether a child or sibling is on the 'at-risk register' (this is changing – but essentially you can check if a child is known to social services)
- Check the notes of siblings and other family members for any suggestion of abuse in the past (child safety trumps confidentiality concerns here)
- Discuss with (depending on age of child) health visitor, named nurse or consultant paediatrician who is responsible for child protection in your area
- Any increase in suspicion should prompt action
- If still not sure, record your concerns clearly and alert other involved members of the practice team
- Review every time the child is seen again in the practice

Special educational needs

What causes of 'failure at school' do GPs and paediatricians encounter?

- Social problems: domestic and peer-related problems (such as bullying or sexual abuse), school absence
- School absence through illness, school refusal, truancy, neglect
- Poor home-schooling
- Educational problems: limited intellect (note that the term 'mental handicap' has been replaced by the term learning disability), attention deficit hyperactivity disorder, autistic spectrum disorder, hearing or vision problems, dyslexia, dyspraxia and other physical handicaps

What legislation supports children with special educational needs?

Since the 1981 Education Act, the education authority is obliged to assess children who may need additional educational provision because of severe or complex difficulties. Following this assessment, a legally binding document is produced: the statement of special educational needs (SSEN). It is reviewed annually, and is drawn up on the basis of an educational psychologist's report, medical report (from hospital and community paediatricians) and reports from other involved professionals such as therapists and a child's nursery or school. The parents are also invited to submit evidence. The child's educational needs and the provision needed to meet them are clearly outlined.

Are children with special needs looked after in special schools?

If possible, children with special educational needs are educated in mainstream schools, with extra help provided in the classroom as needed. There are special schools if mainstream education is not appropriate, and some mainstream schools have specialized language units within them. *Be prepared to talk about advantages and disadvantages in types of schooling*, e.g. large class sizes in state schools.

What other help is there for children with special needs?

Support may be provided by different therapists: occupational therapists, physiotherapists, speech and language therapists and classroom special needs assistants.

Parents can claim disability living allowance (DLA) for children with special needs, including a mobility component from age 5 as well as invalid care allowance (provided they are not in full time employment). There is a care component and a mobility component to the DLA.

Paediatric emergencies: Example – Kawasaki disease

How would you identify Kawasaki disease?

Note: You may also be given signs and symptoms of this disease in a clinical scenario.

The presence of more than five of:

- Fever for > 5 days
- Bilateral non-purulent conjunctivitis
- Polymorphous rash
- Changes in lips and mouth: more reddened, dry or cracked lips
- Strawberry tongue
- Diffuse redness of oropharyngeal mucosa
- Reddened palms or soles or ulcerative oedema of the hands and feet
- Peeling of the skin on the digits of the hands and feet (convalescence)

What are the differential diagnoses of these signs?

- Staphylococcal scalded skin syndrome
- Scarlet fever

- Drug reactions
- Stephens–Johnson syndrome
- Measles

Does a positive swab for streptococcal throat exclude Kawasaki disease?

No.

What is the management of Kawasaki disease?

- Urgently refer to hospital paediatric department
- Early treatment (< 10 days) with intravenous immunoglobulin and aspirin decreases the incidence and severity of complications as well as providing symptomatic relief. Treatment may be given after this time
- Be prepared to talk about the avoidance of aspirin in young children and Reye syndrome in all cases but Kawasaki disease
- Parents should be offered support such as the Kawasaki Support Group (www.patient.co.uk/leaflets/kawasaki_support_group.htm

What are the complications of Kawasaki disease?

- In the acute phase, may cause thromboses, myocardial infarct, dysrhythmias and even death
- Long term –scarring of coronary arteries and accelerated atherosclerosis/ coronary artery disease
- Coronary arteritis leading to coronary aneurysms in 20–30% of untreated patients

Other paediatric emergencies you may be asked to discuss

- Recognition of the seriously unwell child
- Paediatric emergencies – how to estimate a child's weight and fluid requirement
- Management of poisoning
- Management of near-drowning
- Management of burns
- Management of sepsis or meningitis
- Management of diabetic keto-acidosis
- Management of severe croup, epiglottis, asthma or airway obstruction
- Management of the severely injured child

Chronic disease management: Example – paediatric asthma

What are the steps in asthma management for children?

Summary of current BTS/SIGN Guidelines for the management of asthma in children:

For children aged < 5 years:

- Step 1: Use inhaled short acting beta-agonist as needed
- Step 2: Add in inhaled steroid 200–400 μg/day or leukotriene antagonist (such as montelukast) if steroids contraindicated
- Step 3: Children aged 2–5, consider a trial of montelukast and for children aged < 2 consider step 4
- Step 4: Add in oral steroids and refer to respiratory paediatrician

For children aged 5–12 years:

- Step 1: Use inhaled short acting beta agonist as needed
- Step 2: Add in inhaled steroid 200–400 μg/day
- Step 3: Add in long-acting beta agonist (LABA). If there is a good response, continue LABA and increase inhaled steroid to 400 μg/day. If there is no response, stop LABA, increase inhaled steroid to 400 μg/day and consider a trial of montelukast or theophylline
- Step 4: Increase inhaled steroid to 800 μg/day or equivalent
- Step 5: Add in oral steroids and refer to respiratory paediatrician

Are inhaled corticosteroids safe?

Yes, if given at the recommended dose. If the dose is exceeded, then adverse effects may include adrenal suppression. There is no evidence to support preventative low-dose steroid use for episodic viral wheeze.

Which children with asthma need to be referred to a specialist clinic?

- Where there is doubt over the diagnosis
- A child who has a poor response to 800 μg/day of inhaled beclomethasone (or equivalent)
- A child who has reached stage 4 of the BTS/SIGN guideline and should be on other asthma treatments; concordance and drug delivery need careful assessment
- A child who shows a poor response to 400 μg/day of inhaled beclomethasone (or equivalent) and needs add-on therapy that the GP is unfamiliar with

- Young child < 5 years old; uncertainty about drug delivery, this requires (at the very least) access to the expertise of a specialist asthma nurse
- Child under 1 year old; often doubt about diagnosis
- Recurrent admission to hospital which suggests a dangerous pattern of asthma (such patients are often granted 'open access' to children's assessment units or paediatric wards)
- Patients with particularly severe acute asthma, such as needing IV treatment or ICU admission, should always be referred
- Social factors, such as neglect, abuse or poor living conditions

Other chronic diseases you may be asked to discuss

- Diagnosis and management of childhood diabetes
- Causes and management of childhood anaemia
- Diagnosis and management of cystic fibrosis
- Childhood cancer
- Recurrent abdominal pain
- Recurrent headaches

Common paediatric conditions: Example – management of urinary tract infection

What might raise your clinical suspicion of a urinary tract infection (UTI)?

- Must be considered in any small child who is septic or ill, has fever, vomiting or irritability
- May be a cause of poor urine flow
- May be associated with an abdominal or bladder mass
- In a verbal child, a complaint of pain on urination or abdominal pain
- Consider recurrent UTI as a cause of failure to thrive

Would you investigate a suspected UTI before starting treatment?

Antibiotic treatment should not be delayed while awaiting results of microscopy and culture. Recent NICE guidance advocates dipping a urine sample (ideally clean catch) for nitrites and leucocytes if there are moderate symptoms and clinical suspicion (www.nice.org.uk/c6054). All children under 3 months with a first UTI should be referred to paediatrics or paediatric urology (depending on local referral guidelines) for assessment and further investigation. Older children with severe or recurrent UTIs should also be referred.

What further investigations might be offered, and how might you explain them to an anxious parent?

Investigations to consider are ultrasound of the renal tract followed by a micturating cystourethrogram and/or a DMSA (di mercapto succinic acid) scan (the latter to look for renal scarring). A useful leaflet on isotope renal scans can be found on the Royal College of Radiology website (www.rcr.ac.uk/docs/patients/worddocs/radleafnmkidneyf12.doc).

You might explain the need for investigation as follows: 'Appropriate and prompt antibiotic treatment reduces the risk of kidney scarring, which can occur in children as a result of recurrent infections. Young children with urine infections (and children who have severe or recurring infections) need to have investigations done. This is to make sure that they do not have any abnormality of the kidneys, bladder or urinary tract. This is initially an ultrasound scan which may be followed by a test called a "micturating cystourethrogram". Children with renal tract abnormalities need antibiotics to safeguard against infections and kidney damage. Children at risk of kidney scarring will be offered a further test which looks for scarring and is called a DMSA scan.'

What is the treatment for UTI?

- Empirical treatment often depends on local resistance and is usually trimethoprim or nitrofurantoin (consult children's BNF for appropriate age- or weight-related dose)
- Children with renal tract abnormalities or who are awaiting further renal tract investigations should have low-dose prophylaxis (ideally with trimethoprim or nitrofurantoin – see children's BNF)

Other common conditions you may be asked to discuss

- Childhood skin diseases
- Management of gastroenteritis
- Allergy in children
- Earache
- Epistaxis
- Upper respiratory tract infections
- Differentiating minor from serious illness

Paediatric public health: Example – screening

What conditions are screened for in newborn babies and why?

The following is not an exhaustive list:

- **Phenylketonuria (PKU):** The Guthrie test is carried out on blood on filter paper obtained by heel prick. The baby must be on full milk feeds for 3 days before testing. Untreated PKU causes severe learning disability. A low phenylalanine diet prevents the build-up of metabolites which cause brain damage
- **Congenital hypothyroidism:** Analysis of thyroxine and thyroid stimulating hormone, also from blood on filter paper obtained by heel prick – the same sample as PKU testing. If treated early, the child grows and develops normally. Untreated it results in severe learning disability
- **Congenital cataracts:** When looking through an ophthalmoscope, if white light instead of red is reflected from the retina, it suggests a cataract or other ophthalmic pathology. Immediate referral is needed and early treatment prevents permanent visual impairment
- **Cryptorchidism:** If the testes in baby boys are impalpable in the scrotal sac, referral is needed. Undescended testes are at risk of infertility and malignancy. Surgery should be performed before the age of 18 months
- **Developmental dysplasia of the hip:** The Barlow and Ortolani manoeuvres are carried out as part of the neonatal check and at 6 weeks; abnormal findings are confirmed by ultrasound. Early orthopaedic intervention is effective in preventing limp and painful disability from dislocated, subluxed or dysplastic hips
- **Congenital heart disease:** Identification of a heart murmur is the commonest presentation. If cardiac defects at birth are missed, then irreversible cardiopulmonary changes or infective endocarditis may result

What are important criteria for screening tests?

- The condition involved should be an important health problem
- The natural history of the disease should be known
- There should be a recognizable latent or early symptomatic phase
- There should be a test that is easy to perform and interpret
- It should be accurate, reliable, sensitive and specific
- There should be an acceptable, recognized treatment for the disease
- Treatment should be more effective if started early
- There should be a policy on who should be treated
- Diagnosis and treatment should be cost-effective
- Case finding should be continuous

Paediatric public health: Example – immunization

Why do we immunize children?

In developed countries the most beneficial and cost-effective health intervention for the primary prevention of infectious diseases is immunization. One of the primary aims is to provide a population with herd immunity so that the infectious organism cannot survive by chain transmission. Effective herd immunity can only be achieved with immunization rates of around 90% of the population. This is important for the protection of those who cannot be immunized, and because no vaccine is 100% effective.

What is the current immunization schedule in the UK?

- 2 months: diphtheria/tetanus/pertussis/poliomyelitis/haemophilus type B (DTaP/IPV/Hib) (one injection) and pneumococcal vaccine (one injection)
- 3 months: DTaP/IPV/Hib (one injection) and meningococcus group C (MenC) (one injection)
- 4 months: DTaP/IPV/Hib (one injection), MenC (one injection) and pneumococcal vaccine (one injection)
- 12 months: Hib/MenC (one injection)
- 13 months: measles, mumps and rubella (MMR) (one injection) and pneumococcal vaccine (one injection)
- 3 years and 4 months–5 years: DTaP or dTaP (one injection) and MMR (one injection) (reduced dose diphtheria vaccine if aged over 10 or completed primary immunizations in infancy)
- 13–18 years: diphtheria, tetanus and polio (Td/IPV) (one injection)

Up-to-date information on immunization and infectious disease may be found at www.immunisation.nhs.uk.

If a child is allergic to eggs, can they still have the MMR vaccine?

The MMR vaccine may contain small quantities of egg. The concern regarding serious reactions to MMR in children with egg allergy has rarely been borne out when such children have received the vaccine. The vaccine may thus be given. However, if a child has had an anaphylactic reaction to egg, it may be appropriate for the first/next dose of the vaccine to be given in hospital. This is more for parental reassurance than because of the theoretical risk of an adverse reaction. There is no good evidence that skin-testing is helpful to rule out such allergies.

When should immunizations be postponed or avoided?

- Postpone immunizations if a child has a systemic febrile illness, not just 'snuffles' or 'a bit of a cough'. Taking antibiotics is not a contraindication
- Asthma and eczema are not contraindications except in the case of specific allergies (but see above)
- The mother being pregnant again is not a contraindication, but having an immune compromised sibling is a contraindication to live oral polio vaccine
- Vaccination against tuberculosis and other live vaccines should be avoided in HIV-positive children

Other paediatric public health issues you may be asked to discuss

- What is child health surveillance/promotion?
- What do children die from in the UK?
- Childhood obesity
- Role of the school doctor/nurse, health visitor, community midwife

Paediatric surgery: Example – pyloric stenosis

What are the clinical features of pyloric stenosis?

- Projectile vomiting – of curdled and unpleasant-smelling milk, not bile-stained. The baby will be hungry and will feed immediately after vomiting
- Failure to thrive
- Dehydration
- Constipation – due to dehydration. Rabbit pellet stools
- Distended stomach, may have visible peristalsis of the stomach
- 95% have a palpable pyloric mass (like an olive) just below the right costal margin. It is more prominent after vomiting
- May have haematemesis

Are there any special investigations?

Diagnosis is based on clinical findings. A test feed may be done – the baby is given a drink, sat on the parent's lap and the examiner's hand dipped deeply under the liver to find the 'olive-sized' pyloric thickening.

How would you manage this if it presents in A&E or general practice?

The child should be referred acutely to the hospital paediatric department for assessment, metabolic stabilization and subsequent transfer to the care of a paediatric surgeon. The operation performed is a pyloromyotomy.

What is the epidemiology of pyloric stenosis?

This condition usually develops in the first 3–6 weeks of life, and rarely presents in infants over the age of 12 weeks. It is commonest in first-born, male children.

Other paediatric surgical conditions you may be asked to discuss

- Appendicitis
- Abdominal wall hernias
- Neck lumps
- Transplant patients
- Intussusception – recognition and management
- Circumcision and urological problems
- Congenital abnormalities requiring urgent referral

Child development: Example – flat feet in toddlers

Scenario

A mother has brought her 2-year-old girl to the GP because she is flat footed and her feet seem to point inward a little when she runs. Standing on tiptoe (which she does not do for long) there is no convincing medial arch.

How would you advise her?

This example serves to illustrate that anything which presents to GPs may be used in this exam. Pes planus (or flat foot) is where the arch of the foot is low. There may be valgus and eversion foot deformities. The most important advice is that flat feet are normal in children who are learning to walk. The medial arch develops over the next few years. If flat feet persist, no action is necessary provided that the medial arch of the foot restores itself on tiptoe.

The mother wants to know if there is anything which she can do to help her daughter develop healthy feet

Some research shows that children who are allowed to go barefoot until the age of 6 years have healthier feet. Some GPs suggest exercises to produce the arch; these involve the child flexing their forefoot and toes, 'like a crawly caterpillar!'

Would anything make you concerned in such a circumstance?

High arches in a small child who has a clumsy gait might raise suspicion of cerebral palsy or muscular dystrophy. Any other signs of ataxia might raise suspicion of neurological disease or a posterior fossa tumour.

Other child development issues you may be asked to discuss:

- Fields of child development
- Hearing assessment
- Normal/abnormal milestones
- Learning difficulties
- Communication difficulties
- Movement disorders

Important neonatal problems: Example – jaundice

What causes jaundice in newborn babies? Is it common?

Jaundice is benign in most babies – it is due to problems with bilirubin metabolism and clearance. Approximately 50% of term and 80% of preterm babies become jaundiced.

When should you take notice of jaundice?

Jaundice is regarded as pathological if it occurs within 24 hours of birth or more than 3 weeks after birth. Some babies have clinically obvious jaundice for> 10 days after birth. Certain risk factors (Rh incompatibility, birth trauma, infection, polycythaemia, hypothyroidism or poor feeding) may lead to high plasma bilirubin levels with a risk of neurotoxicity and kernicterus. A raised conjugated bilirubin in a jaundiced child suggests biliary obstruction and should be referred immediately to the paediatric department. The paediatrician may refer the child on to a paediatric specialist liver unit.

Can plasma bilirubin concentration be reliably estimated by clinical examination?

No. If risk factors are present, bilirubin levels should be tested on a venous or capillary blood sample and/or transcutaneous bilirubinometry.

What is the treatment of clinically significant jaundice?

Treatment is with phototherapy with blue light. Very high levels may require an exchange transfusion.

What is breast-milk jaundice?

This is the commonest reason for jaundice lasting beyond 10 days (unconjugated hyperbilirubinaemia). Mothers can mostly be reassured that it usually resolves by 6 weeks but may continue for 3 months. The jaundice disappears if breast feeding is stopped, but this action is only advised in exceptional circumstances.

Other neonatal problems you may be asked to discuss

- Routine care at delivery and neonatal resuscitation
- Group B Streptococcus (GBS) in pregnancy and signs of GBS septicaemia in infancy
- Respiratory distress
- Congenital cyanotic heart disease
- Feeding problems and hypoglycaemia in infancy
- Low birth weight and prematurity
- The neonatal examination and problems which may be picked up

Further reading

Beattie M, Clark A, Smith A. *Short Cases for the Paediatric Membership.* Knutsford: PasTest, 2004: p. 239–41.

Bellman M, Kennedy N, eds. *Paediatrics and Child Health. A Textbook for the DCH.* Edinburgh: Churchill Livingstone, 2000, p. 341–2.

Bellman M, Peile E. *The Normal Child*. Edinburgh: Churchill Livingstone, 2006: p. 199–200 (Childhood immunizations).

Cartwright S, Godlee C. Urinary tract infections in children. In: Nagawan B, ed. *Churchill's Pocketbook of General Practice*, 3rd edn. Edinburgh: Churchill Livingstone, 2005: p. 82–3.

Collier J, Longmore M, Brunsden M, eds. Orthopaedics and trauma. In: *Oxford Handbook of Clinical Specialties*, 7th edn. Oxford: Oxford University Press, 2007: p. 672.

Elliman D, Bedford H. Parents' immunization questions answered. *Pulse* Jan 2008.

Huertas-Ceballos A. Common problems in preterm babies. In: Bellman M, Peile E, eds. *The Normal Child*. Edinburgh: Churchill Livingstone, 2006: p. 24–7.

Le Fanu J. Wrongful diagnosis of child abuse – a master theory. *J R Soc Med* 2005;**98**:249–54.

Miall M, Rudolf M, Levene M. Screening and surveillance tests. In: *Paediatrics at a Glance*, 2nd edn. Oxford: Blackwell Science, 2007: p. 49.

Mori R, Lakhanpaul M, Verrier-Jones K. Diagnosis and management of urinary tract infections in children: Summary of NICE Guidance. *BMJ* 2007;**335**: 395–7.

National Institute for Health and Clinical Excellence. *Urinary tract infection in children: Diagnosis, treatment and long-term management*. London: NICE, 2007. www.nice.org.uk

Royal College of General Practitioners. *The Role of Primary Care in the Protection of Children from Abuse and Neglect: A Position Paper*. London: RCGP, 2002. www.rcgp.org.uk

Rudolf M, Levene M. *Paediatrics and Child Health*, 2nd edn. Oxford: Blackwell Science, 2006: p. 228–9, 324–5.

Simon C, O'Reilly K, Proctor R, Buckmaster J. *Emergencies in Primary Care*. Oxford: Oxford University Press, 2007.

Townshend J, Hails S, McKean M. Clinical review: Management of asthma in children. *BMJ* 2007;**335**:253–7.

Anchor statement:

	Expected Standard/ CLEAR PASS	PASS
RAPPORT	Full greeting and introduction Clarifies role and agrees aims and objectives Good eye contact and posture. Perceived to be actively listening (nod, etc.) with verbal and non-verbal cues Appropriate level of confidence Empathetic nature. Putting parent/child at ease	Adequately performed but not fully fluent in conducting interview
INFORMATION GATHERING	Asks clear questions. Patient and examiner can hear and understand fully Mixture of open and closed style Avoids jargon Allows parent/child sufficient time to speak Picks up verbal and non-verbal cues Verifies and summarizes parent/child history	Questions reasonable and cover all essential issues but may omit occasional relevant but less important points Overall approach structured Appropriate style of questioning responsive to parent/child Summarizes history
INFORMATION GIVING	Information given is accurate Language is understandable to parent/child Knowledge base for information is appropriate for F2 doctor (or equivalent) with paediatric training	Accurate information except in minor detail Language is generally appropriate for parent/child's level of understanding Knowledge base poor in minor areas

Communication skills

BARE FAIL	CLEAR FAIL	UNACCEPTABLE
Incomplete or hesitant greeting and introduction Inadequate identification of role, aims and objectives Poor eye contact and posture. Not perceived to be actively listening (nod, etc.) with verbal and non-verbal cues Does not show appropriate level of confidence, empathetic nature or putting parent/child at ease	Significant components omitted or not achieved	Dismissive of parent/child concerns Fails to put parent or child at ease Lack of civility or politeness Inappropriate manner including flippancy
Misses relevant information which if known would make a difference to the management of the problem Excessive use of closed instead of open questions Uses medical jargon occasionally Misses verbal or non-verbal cues Summary inaccurate/incomplete	Asks closed questions instead of open questions Questions poorly comprehended by parent/child Inappropriate use of medical jargon Inappropriately interrupts parent/child. Hasty approach Does not seek views of parent or child Poorly structured interview	Shows no regard for parent or child's feelings Rudeness or arrogance No verification or summarising
Some inaccurate information given Language difficult for parent/child to understand Knowledge base poor in major areas	Much information inaccurate but not dangerous Language inappropriate for parent/child to understand Knowledge base generally poor	Dangerous or grossly inaccurate information Language impossible for parent/child to understand Knowledge base below that expected for any qualified doctor

7 Communication skills

There are two communication skills stations, each lasting 5 minutes. As with the nMRCGP examination, the relative lack of reliable child actors means that these stations will often involve dealing with a parent, carer or healthcare professional *in the absence of a child.* You may be asked to talk to a real parent and/or child, a health professional or a member of the public. A telephone conversation, e.g. with a parent/doctor/professional, may be included.

The scenarios in this chapter test clinical knowledge and different aspects of communication and applied knowledge – DCH candidates may use scenarios such as these in timed role-play, and generate further role play based on any issues that they may encounter or have difficulty with. The sample scenarios below have been subdivided in to three sections: post-admission counselling, child health advice and advice about a baby. These aim to reflect the three main types of advice concerning children that may be requested of a GP. *Remember that this exam is increasingly aimed at GPs rather than paediatricians, who are encouraged to do MRCPCH instead.*

Each of the scenarios could be expected to be tackled by a DCH candidate within the allotted 5 minutes, and points to cover/issues to consider are also given. Some of the scenarios might easily form the basis of a 10-minute consultation in general practice. (The author of this chapter has also encountered some of the scenarios as 'emergency consultations' in practice.) However, candidates are expected to do their best in 5 minutes – *it is possible to pass the station without completing all possible items provided that the candidate closes the interview and arranges appropriate follow-up with the actor.*

According to the Royal College of Paediatrics and Child Health, there are six main patterns of communication scenario (www.rcpch/Examinations/DCH/DCH-Clinical-Structure Candidate Guidenotes):

- **Information giving** (e.g. please tell this parent about the diagnosis)
- **Consent** (e.g. please explain why you need to do a lumbar puncture with a view to obtaining consent)
- **Critical incident** (e.g. please talk to the parent of the child who has been given the wrong drug)
- **Ethics** (e.g. please discuss the problem as Anna has refused to have any blood tests)
- **Education** (e.g. please explain the situation to a healthcare professional so that she can deal with it)
- **Explain the use of common medical devices**. A manikin or model may be used in such a station. There will be a specific task that a GP would be expected to be able to undertake (e.g. explain how to use a steroid nasal spray, a salbutamol inhaler or a peak expiratory flow meter)

You need to be aware of some generic explaining and negotiating skills for the OSCE, even though this may appear to be obvious advice:

- Introduce yourself and establish the identity of the person(s) you are addressing
- Establish the reason for the interview: Why has the patient come to see you? It may be useful to recap: Do they understand what has taken place so far?
- Remember that ideas, concerns and expectations (ICE) are important
- Try not to interrupt a parent who is telling you about the problem; they may well give you more of the answer and it is considered rude to butt in!
- Explain what you need to but allow the person in front of you to express their views
- Discuss pros, cons and alternatives of any course of action
- Put parents at ease and avoid being judgemental at all costs
- Avoid jargon; explain terms if necessary. Remember to summarize and recognize opportunities to check understanding/offer to answer questions
- If relevant, offer some written material such as a leaflet or website address
- Offer further/continuing support and keep further meetings open
- Where parents are having difficulties with small children, or you have any concern for the welfare of the child, a follow-up home visit (for example) by the health visitor can be arranged
- Close the meeting, thank the ‘parent/child’ for coming and say goodbye
- No matter how good your communication skills are, some clinical knowledge is needed to manage these stations

Post-admission counselling

General advice

Parents whose children are discharged from the A&E or the paediatric ward are often told to 'see their GP' for follow-up. It is useful to spend a minute or two 'data gathering' from the parent. Recap on what has taken place and ask what advice they were given on admission and discharge.

> **Scenario 1**
>
> Mrs Jones has come to see you because her daughter Jane, aged 3, was recently admitted to A&E with a febrile convulsion.

As with all such consultations, a recap on what has happened will yield useful material for discussion.

The main aims of the consultation are to: reassure the parents about the benign nature of the disorder; and educate them about prognosis, causes and what to do if it recurs, so that they are not overly anxious about febrile illness in children.

- Febrile seizures are the most common seizure disorder. They are defined as occurring between 6 months and 6 years of age
- Children generally have a normal cognitive and developmental outcome
- They recur in a third of children and are associated with a low risk of epilepsy

Assess risk factors for epilepsy: complex febrile seizure, neurological abnormality and family history of epilepsy

Was Jane's seizure complex?

Complex seizures are defined by at least one of: duration longer than 15 minutes, multiple seizures within 24 hours and focal features.

Where a seizure lasts longer than 5 minutes, an ambulance should be called (or local doctor/paramedic in remote locations). If seizures recur before a child has returned to normal, they need to be sent to hospital and rectal diazepam or buccal midazolam needs to be given. Where a child has recurrent febrile convulsions, parents can be instructed on the administration of rectal diazepam.

Paracetamol and ibuprofen are often useful in relieving the discomfort of a febrile child, but there is no direct evidence that rigorous reduction of temperature reduces the recurrence of seizures. Tepid sponging is another method of controlling temperature which gives parents a greater sense of participation in the care of a febrile child. Tepid sponging does appear to work but the evidence is not spectacular.

Scenario 2

Mr Pope has brought his 2-year-old son, Alexander, to see you. Alexander has had vomiting and diarrhoea for 2 days. At the local Emergency Medical Department they were told 'to visit you the following day'.

Establish what Mr Pope was told about Alexander's diarrhoea, what advice he was given and what the symptoms were attributed to? You may wish briefly to recap on the symptoms:

- What is the nature of the stool (bloody? watery?) and how often is Alexander passing a motion?
- Is he passing less urine? When was the last wet nappy? Has he lost any weight?
- How often and for how long has he been vomiting? Is he taking fluids or paracetamol?
- Does he have any major health problems or previous hospital admissions?
- Has anyone else at home been sick?
- Has there been any change in his diet?
- Any recent travel

This scenario (if there are no worrying symptoms) is about reassuring the parent, whilst laying an appropriate safety net should things get worse:

- Gastroenteritis is the most common cause of diarrhoea and vomiting. As it is mostly caused by viruses, antibiotics are of no use
- Treatment is supportive, and the symptoms usually resolve within a week. Paracetamol is advocated more for symptoms of pain distress or lethargy rather than for a fever per se
- If the parents are worried, they can always bring him back or call for help if he is poorly out of hours. If he becomes unresponsive/unrouseable or has a fit, displays fear of the light, abnormal posture or any symptom that makes his parents very worried, they should consider taking him straight to the nearest A&E department
- Oral rehydration solution (Dioralyte) is available over the counter at chemists

- Sometimes children with diarrhoea may develop transient lactose intolerance
- Breast feeds should be continued for babies with vomiting and diarrhoea

The history and counselling above is for acute diarrhoea. Chronic diarrhoea in an infant is also a potential scenario which might bring a parent to see a GP. Try to differentiate between the four main causes of chronic diarrhoea: toddler diarrhoea, secondary cow's milk/lactose intolerance, coeliac disease and cystic fibrosis.

Scenario 3

Mrs Papas has come to see you because her son Nicholas, aged 6, was recently admitted overnight with an anaphylactoid reaction to peanuts

It may be useful to recap on what has happened:

- What was done in hospital, what medications were prescribed (is he taking Piriton and prednisolone?)
- What follow-up has been advised?
- Did Nicholas have a previous history of atopy, such as eczema, asthma or hayfever? (Most fatal reactions to food occur in people with asthma. Asthma should be optimally controlled.)

In IgE-mediated food allergy (such as the above) common triggers include eggs, milk, peanuts and fish (including seafood); less common triggers include fruit, vegetables and tree nuts. Reactions typically occur within minutes of ingesting the food. They are typically local: angioedema (swelling), perioral itching, laryngeal oedema (sore throat and noisy breathing), and systemic: urticarial rash, soreness of eyes and nose, wheeze, diarrhoea and vomiting and, in some cases, anaphylaxis.

Has Nicholas had any previous investigations for food allergy? Ask about food-specific skin prick tests. For those in whom true food allergy is suspected, or for whom the diagnosis cannot be safely excluded, serum-specific IgE tests to the foods implicated can be performed. Indiscriminate testing is not recommended as tests have low specificity.

Attempt to distinguish true allergy from food intolerance. In food intolerance, symptoms are typically non-specific, making it difficult to establish a temporal relationship between food and symptoms, and at times the foods may be well tolerated.

IgE-mediated food allergy will require complete avoidance of the provoking foods. Help from a paediatric dietician with detailed written strategies on food avoidance is useful. Advise scrutiny of the ingredients on packaged cakes and ready meals.

Nicholas needs to be referred to an allergy specialist and ought to have the serum-specific IgE tests while waiting to be assessed (the paediatricians may already have arranged this). Advise the patient/parents that the food triggers should be avoided completely.

For patients who have had life-threatening symptoms, prescribe a self-administered epinephrine auto-injector (Epipen). Patients/parents will need a detailed written plan advising them when and how to use this. The school (alert the school nurse) may also need advice and training. Many hospital resuscitation officers offer training sessions for parents following an anaphylactic reaction in their child.

Offer written information on allergy and anaphylaxis; websites such as www.anaphylaxis.org may offer further information. A Medicalert bracelet may also be useful (www.medicalert.org.uk).

Scenario 4

Mrs Smith has just been seen in A&E with 2-year-old Britanny who has accidentally swallowed some cleaning products. She was in A&E 2 months ago after her 1-year-old burned herself with a cup of tea. Please talk to her about accident prevention.

Introduce yourself and put the parent at ease.
Acknowledge how difficult it can be looking after toddlers. Does she have any help?
Do not blame her; a non-judgemental attitude helps.

Offer to give her some advice to make her home safer. Aged 2 most children are walking and curious about their environment. This is a potentially accident prone time! Most accidents (adults and children) occur in the living room, followed by the kitchen.

- Is the child adequately supervised, especially when eating or in an area where they can roam and are free to fall or encounter a hazard?
- Are medicines kept locked away and out of reach?
- Are locks fitted on cupboards where knives, medications and cleaning products are stored? Stairgates and plug-socket covers?
- Are small objects which could be swallowed or aspirated out of reach?
- Are electrical flexes out of reach of curious little hands?
- Are hot pans/stoves, kettles/irons and their cables, and hot drinks out of reach?

- Water safety – care with baths: testing water temperature, not leaving unattended
- Not smoking (especially indoors) and safety in the bedroom – back to sleep campaign for babies
- Road safety, car seats, seatbelts

Offer contact with the health visitor to visit and check her home/offer advice. Ongoing support may be provided by the GP or health visitor, and childcare assistance possibilities explored. Useful books, e.g. *Birth to Five*, can be offered.

Ask if there are any questions and attempt to answer these. Offer a follow-up visit.

Child health advice

> **Scenario 1**
>
> You have been asked to talk to Mr Smith about the MMR vaccination for his boy Johnny, aged 18 months. Though his wife is keen to proceed, Mr Smith has an autistic son, aged 10, by a previous marriage.

Warning: Do not become too distracted by issues of parental responsibility while this discussion is taking place. Though the father has parental responsibility, this should be a shared decision. He probably just wants to discuss his concerns. If a parent or third party were actively seeking a treatment for a child and the other parent were known to be objecting to it, this would prompt discussion of parental responsibility and the best interests of the child.

General advice

Ultimately a parent may choose to disagree with you. If so, offer information and the opportunity to return for further discussion.

Introduce yourself and put him at ease, 'What can I do for you today?'
Listen to and acknowledge his ideas and concerns, 'What in particular concerns you about the MMR vaccine? What have you read? Do you have personal experience of children with autism?'

Do not be judgmental or coercive. 'It is your decision to do what you feel is best for your child.'

Points to address

Scientific evidence linking the MMR vaccine to autism is lacking. The number of cases of autism has been increasing since 1979. There has been no sudden increase with the introduction of the MMR vaccine in the UK in 1988. Several large European studies have found no association between MMR and autism.

Autism is commonly diagnosed after 18 months of age as children start to talk and interact. It has a genetic component and associated neurological abnormalities have been seen to start in the womb. MMR is given twice: at 13 months and at preschool entry to 'boost' immunity, so parents may sometimes associate the onset of autism with the MMR. The original paper in the *Lancet* by Wakefield et al described a case series of only 12 children, failed to take the above points into account and has now been discredited.

Known side effects of MMR: 10% develop fever, malaise and a rash 5–21 days after the first vaccination; 3% develop painful joints. Special vaccination precautions are needed in children with severe anaphylactic reactions to egg or chronic severe asthma.

Single vaccines: There is no evidence of any benefit. The US, Canada and 38 European countries use MMR. Single vaccines mean three times the distress, three visits, risk of febrile reactions, longer time taken to establish immunity – and a longer period where the child is unprotected. The single vaccines are not available on the NHS – parents will have to pay.

Dangers of non-vaccination: Measles can cause death, pneumonia, deafness and a slow relentless form of encephalitis (subacute sclerosing panencephalitis). Mumps may result in meningitis, pancreatitis and sterility from orchitis. The babies of pregnant women exposed to rubella may suffer congenital rubella syndrome – deafness, blindness, heart problems and brain damage. Measles is contagious. Every child with measles infects 15 others. If < 96% of children are immunized (as is now the case in the UK), then an epidemic may occur.

There is a great deal of information to give so Mr Smith may need to come back after having thought about what he has been told. You can offer an information leaflet/website suggestions such as the government website www.nmrthefacts.nhs.uk (which refers to inflammatory bowel disease and autism). Summarize and ask Mr Smith if he has any questions.

Remember there is not much time – keep your advice simple, explore concerns and offer a follow-up appointment, ideally with both parents present. There is no need to refer to an expert except for special vaccination precautions, or if there are ongoing parental concerns.

Scenario 2

Mrs Hardwicke would like something for her 8-year-old boy, Jeremy, to 'help him go'. He's been struggling to go to the toilet once every few days. It is now quite painful, he cries at the thought of going to the toilet and his tummy is starting to get tender and bloated.

Ask about: Jeremy's diet and fluid intake, his previous bowel habit, and how the parents and child are coping. Does he ever have any accidents with his bowels or bladder? You would like to see Jeremy to 'feel his tummy'.

Acute constipation is caused by:

- Dehydration – fever, hot environment, not drinking
- Bowel obstruction – are and sometimes due to congenital malformations, more likely to present as an acute abdomen
- A change of diet or environment (such as a decrease in dietary fibre and fluids)

Laxatives may be required; Movicol is currently 'in fashion' (can use lactulose)

Chronic constipation can be:

- Functional – common with disabled children
- Secondary to withholding, such as with an anal fissure

These do respond to treatment with diet and/or laxatives and bowel training. Be aware that chronic constipation may present with overflow diarrhoea or soiling.

Management:

- Examination of the abdomen, looking for anal fissures or neurological causes
- Evacuation: diet, laxatives (lactulose/Movicol), rarely enemas, even more rarely manual disimpaction under anaesthesia
- Maintenance with diet/laxative for 3–6 months, allocating regular times a day when a child sits on the toilet for 10–15 minutes
- Following return to normal: vigilance and early use of treatment at the first sign of hard stool
- If the child is deliberately soiling in inappropriate places (encopresis), then refer to a child psychiatrist

Advice for parent (www.childhoodconstipation.com):

- Do not let your child wait to do a poo
- Give your child enough time so that they do not feel rushed. Set time aside each day for your child to sit on the toilet, ideally after meals
- Make going to the toilet fun, with treats such as a favourite book or blowing bubbles
- If 'it hurts to poo,' they can stop and try again later
- Lots of active play will increase bowel activity
- Try to include a variety of high-fibre foods in the family's diet, as well as dried fruit, fruit with skin on and vegetables – especially green beans and lentils (can be puréed for babies)
- Encourage your child to drink 6–8 glasses of water or fruit juice per day (avoid caffeinated fizzy drinks)

Scenario 3

Mrs Freeley has come to discuss her son, Peter, aged 8. He wets the bed most nights. He has been dry during the day since he was 4. The only treatment which he has ever had was desmopressin for a sleepover at a friend's house, aged 7. In 6 months the family are going on a long holiday to Canada.

Bed-wetting (nocturnal enuresis) is a common issue for young children: 10% of 5-year-olds and 5% of 10-year-olds wet the bed. Enquire into the family circumstances; this may illuminate the cause or affect management.

History is crucial: Has the child ever been dry? If the answer is yes, then a cause needs to be found: this might be a urine infection or a first presentation of diabetes. It could be a manifestation of bullying or abuse.

Is the child dry at night or dry during the day? Specific treatment is often unnecessary for those under the age of 7 years who have never been dry. About 1% of children with wetting have an organic problem. Daytime urinary symptoms in a bed-wetting child suggest an underlying bladder dysfunction. Diabetes, UTI, constipation and structural anomalies should be excluded.

It should be emphasized that once a physical problem is ruled out, Peter has a very good chance of achieving dry nights in the long term. However, lasting benefit will require motivation by both Peter and his family. A further appointment for the parents and their son is mandatory, as well as referral if feasible to the local enuresis clinic. Printed information helps. The ERIC website is a valuable resource for parents worried about their child's continence: http://www.eric.org.uk.

Enuresis alarms are effective and safe, but do require several months of continual use and may disrupt family sleep. Desmopressin improves bedwetting in the short term, but relapse occurs on stopping without other management. Oral desmopressin may be an option for travel, short holidays and sleepovers. As of April 2007, this indication for desmopressin as a nasal spray is no longer recommended, but tablets are still in use. Imipramine (an antidepressant) is no longer recommended because of a high risk of serious adverse effects in overdose. (See Chapter 6 for common treatment options for nocturnal enuresis.)

Scenario 4

Mrs Thomas would like some advice about her 3-year-old, John. While bathing him, she has noticed that his foreskin is not retractile. He seems obsessed with his penis and his childminder has noticed him playing with himself. Should he have a circumcision?

The foreskin is normally not retractile for the first year, and is non-retractile for 60% of 6-year-olds because of physiological adhesions, which resolve on their own. Retraction of the foreskin may be attempted in 6-year-old boys for hygiene purposes, but not to tear adhesions, which can cause scarring. Circumcision is rarely medically indicated, and there is intense debate over whether cultural circumcision is an abuse of children's rights.

You can offer to see John. In all likelihood his obsession with his own genitals is normal and will pass – if it does not, further discussion is needed. Circumcision is reserved for especially troublesome symptoms:

- Recurrent balanitis (> 3 attacks, usual treatment with antibiotic ointment only)
- Phimosis (uncommon), only consider circumcision if difficulty voiding (ballooning is not an indication). Almost all physiological tightness of the foreskin resolves on its own
- Paraphimosis should be reduced as soon as possible (reduce swelling of glans with ice) and, if this is not possible, the child should be referred as an emergency
- Excessive amounts of (redundant) foreskin causing irritation and discomfort

Doctors who perform circumcisions should be able to take informed consent from, ideally, both parents and to manage postoperative pain (main complication). Circumcision of children who are still in nappies can result in ulceration of the urethral meatus and subsequent urethral strictures.

In all likelihood, reassurance and some printed information will suffice unless there is a specific indication.

Scenario 5

Mrs Killpatrick has booked an emergency appointment with you. While cleaning Kirsten's, her 15-year-old daughter's, room she has found a used packet of Microgynon 30 ED. She is distressed and angry. Your notes show that a partner in the surgery felt that Kirsten was competent to make the decision, and Kirsten asked that her parents were not informed.

Contraception, Young People and Confidentiality: The GMC guidance '0–18, which came into force on 13th October 2007, is *mandatory reading*. The following advice is distilled from the GMC guidance.

In this case you are 'not allowed' to discuss any part of Kirsten's health record without her explicit consent. The exception would be if you suspected abusive or seriously harmful sexual activity (presumed so in any child under the age of 13). However, you can discuss Mrs Killpatrick's concerns and worries, talk to Kirsten's usual doctor and find out from Mrs Killpatrick whether she suspects an abusive sexual relationship (essentially the discussion you might have in the absence of the notes and any foreknowledge of the absent patient). 'Has Kirsten's behaviour changed recently? Is she doing OK at school? Has she got a new group of friends or a boyfriend? Have you had any recent discussions with her about what's going on in her life?'

Stating that you did not prescribe her the pill may itself be considered a breech of confidentiality.

Information should be shared about sexual activity if:

- A young person too immature to understand or consent
- Big differences in age, maturity or power between sexual partners
- A young person's sexual partner having a position of trust
- Force or the threat of force, emotional or psychological pressure, bribery or payment, to engage in sex or to keep it secret
- Drugs or alcohol used to influence a young person to have sex, when otherwise they would not
- Sex involving a person known to the police or child protection agencies as a child abuser

Contraception, abortion and advice and treatment for sexually transmitted infections may be given without parental knowledge to children under the age of 16 years provided that:

- They understand the advice and its implications
- You cannot persuade them to tell or allow you to tell the parents
- There is likelihood of sex without treatment
- Physical or mental health will suffer without advice or treatment
- It is in 'best interests' to receive advice or treatment without parental knowledge

The GMC advice is that consultations should be kept confidential even if treatment or advice has not been provided. At age 16 it is legally presumed that young people have the ability to make decisions about the treatment and advice they receive.

Scenario 6

Mrs Smith is worried about her 15-year-old daughter, Sarah. Sarah has been doing less well at school, and yesterday Mrs Smith found some cannabis hidden in her daughter's room. Mrs Smith confesses to having 'smoked dope' in the 70s , but is really worried that Sarah will want to try more dangerous drugs. Sarah does not know her mother is seeing you.

Remember: you cannot divulge information about a third party, although you may have to take action if there is a duty of care to someone who lacks capacity.

You are unable to discuss Sarah's health record in the absence of explicit consent from Sarah and unless there is compelling reason. You may begin by asking Mrs Smith what her concerns are and finding out more. She may just want to air her worries and you can provide her with some facts and sources of support and advice. A useful website is www.talktofrank.com. The 'Talk to Frank' helpline number is 0800 776600 (UK only).

How is Sarah behaving? What effect is this having at home, with friends or at school? Are there any family, interpersonal or emotional problems? Is there a previous or family history of mental health problems, or is she merely a typical 'troubled' teenager? What does she do with her friends, and who does she confide in?

You may suggest that it is appropriate to invite Sarah for an appointment. Any suggestion that she is not competent or mentally ill should prompt a desire to seek senior advice (and advice from a medical defence provider). Warn Mrs Smith that you may need to talk to Sarah alone if they come together.

Cannabis use is common amongst teenagers in the UK: 10% of under-16s reported using it in 2006. Its possession is still a criminal offence, which may result in confiscation and prosecution. Heavy cannabis use does increase the risk of schizophrenia and depression in susceptible individuals, especially if there is a family history of mental illness. Also, today's cannabis is much stronger than that available in the 60s and 70s. Smoking cannabis adds smoking-related risks.

Acknowledge Mrs Smith's concerns – many do believe that cannabis use leads to abuse of other substances and other problems. This is partly because drug use is more common in 11–16-year-olds with ADHD, truancy, depression and other psychosocial disorders. It is also because the drug affects education, work and driving skills, and may lead to less awareness of personal safety, such as vigilance about sexual intercourse or trying other drugs. It can affect the developing brain. Side effects do include paranoia, confusion and anxiety.

Explore Mrs Smith's ideas, concerns and expectations in this consultation. Let her know that you are willing to explore local sources of support if necessary, and that you are willing to broach the topic with Sarah at her next consultation.

Scenario 7

Mrs Doyle has made an urgent appointment to see you regarding her son Len, aged 7. During a recent wheezy episode following a viral illness, one of the partners at your surgery prescribed a steroid inhaler. She is worried that this will make his bones brittle, stunt his growth and make him aggressive.

Be aware of the latest BTS Guidelines for Asthma in children under 5 and children aged 5–12 (see Chapter 6).

Len needs his management reviewed. There is no evidence to support preventative low-dose corticosteroid use in viral wheeze. You may need briefly to recap to find out if asthma is suspected. Was the medication prescribed for prophylaxis or for the acute episode only? Look for any suspicion of alternative diagnoses: is there wet cough, stridor, voice change or weight loss? Len may not yet be measuring peak flows, but may be able to start this soon.

Assess control of wheeze: is there wheeze or cough? Are nights distressed, has there been absence from school or interference with play and activities? Assess the frequency of use of his short-acting bronchodilator (blue inhaler), oral steroids or emergency consultations. Ask about possible triggers? If a pattern suggestive of asthma has emerged, then Len needs regular review to assess inhaler technique and measure his growth. Over time an individual asthma

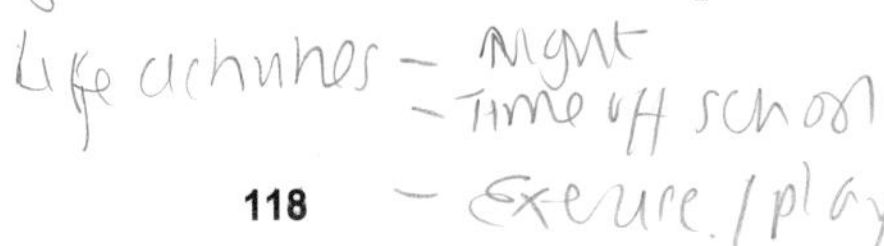

management plan needs to be negotiated, including times when medication should be increased and when Len needs to be seen.

Evaluate Mrs Doyle's ideas, concerns and expectations surrounding asthma. Does she understand the role of the 'reliever' and 'preventer'? It is important for the development of a growing boy to have an improved exercise tolerance and lung development, and growth may be assisted by an inhaled bronchodilator and/or steroid. Inhaled steroids are given at a very low dose. They are safe provided that they are used appropriately. Used excessively, inhaled steroids may cause problems such as adrenal suppression, which is why supervision over time by a doctor or practice nurse is important. However, osteoporosis is associated with long term oral steroid use. You may reassure her about the aggression and stunting of growth.

Note: It is also worth having a working knowledge of the diagnosis and management of allergic rhinoconjunctivitis in children, and the role of steroid and decongestant nasal sprays.

Scenario 8

Ms Shzerpanik would like to obtain some 'strong steroid cream' for her daughter Laura, aged 2. Laura has had some patches of rough dry skin behind her knees and in front of her elbows. She also wants to know about medicated bubble baths.

A brief recap and history may be useful, as will a brief explanation of the implicit problem. Is there a family history of asthma, eczema or hayfever? Did Laura have eczema on her face or nappy rash as a baby? What has the family tried so far? Have there been any changes at home or any new pets?

Eczema is a longstanding inflammation of the skin, often associated with a family history. It causes intense itching, is made worse by scratching and mainly affects the face, and elbow and knee flexures in toddlers. About 12–15% of children are affected by allergic eczema (avoid the use of 'atopy' in consultations as you will have to waste time explaining it). The good news is that three-quarters of children grow out of it by the age of 15 years. Scratching and rubbing actually cause most of the clinical signs. Sleep may be affected and children with eczema are sometimes hyperactive. Untreated it can cause skin damage, which sometimes results in teasing and bullying at school, and in toddlers it may even affect growth (if severe). Eczema is prone to infection with bacteria and with certain viruses – if parents suspect this they should bring their child to the GP to be checked.

Skin-prick tests or blood tests for specific allergens may be useful only if specific triggers for allergy are suspected. If the rash ever looks red or sore and infected, then swabs may be useful to check for infection to guide the use of antibiotics.

General measures

- By now you will have explained what eczema is and offered a printed leaflet from Patient UK, the British Association of Dermatologists or the National Eczema Society (www.eczema.org). The good prognosis will have been mentioned
- Children should wear loose cotton clothing and avoid wool (which irritates) and excessive heat
- Nails should be kept short
- Cats and dogs tend to make eczema worse; ideally keep the child away from them
- House dust mite is a factor but is difficult completely to remove from the home
- Avoid soaps and bubble baths (these can be drying and irritant, especially if scented)
- First-line treatment is with emollients. Regular use of aqueous cream and emulsifying ointments (and as soap substitutes) may help. Mrs Shzerpanik could also use a bath oil emollient
- An antihistamine may help, especially with itching at night
- Second-line treatment is with topical steroids – doctors should prescribe the least potent effective ointment (e.g. 1% hydrocortisone BD). Stronger doses may be needed in flare-ups
- Treat secondary infection promptly
- Consider dermatology referral once the above have been tried without success

Should Laura avoid wheat?

Some children with atopic eczema and a history which is suggestive of food allergy (such as mouth rashes, stomach aches, relationship between a foodstuff and symptoms) should avoid the offending food. Dietary exclusion may also be tried when eczema is resistant to other therapy, but the child should have been referred by this point. A paediatric dietician should be involved to make sure the offending food is excluded but dietary deficiencies are avoided in a growing child.

> ### Scenario 9
> Mrs Brown has come to see you about her daughter, Georgina, aged 10. The school nurse has voiced concerns that Georgina is significantly overweight (BMI 35). She is being teased and bullied.

Remember: plump children are often seen as 'healthy children'; a parent's desire to feed their child is often perceived as instinctive. You may be faced with denial that there is any problem.

- Obesity is an increasing problem in developed countries
- Overweight children are more likely to be socially isolated and have psychological problems
- Being overweight is associated with other lifestyle-related diseases in adulthood, including heart disease, diabetes, asthma and cancers of the breast and bowels, as well as osteoarthritis
- Overweight children are twice as likely to be overweight adults, and this likelihood is higher if a parent is overweight or there is a relapse following weight loss

Five minutes is enough time to explore the mother's concerns and expectation, and to provide education on what further appointments will involve. You should arrange to see the mother and daughter together, weigh Georgina and plot her weight and height against an appropriate paediatric centile chart. Because of the changes in childhood adiposity, BMI should be interpreted with caution.

You should ask permission to get information from the school as needed. Georgina is still growing, so she must aim to maintain a steady weight or to reduce the speed at which she puts on weight. There is little evidence that 'weight loss' diets and medication actually work.

The earlier the intervention, the higher will be the likelihood of success. Though obesity can have a genetic component, it is far more likely that the problem is one of a mismatch between food intake and physical activity. Eating patterns are often set by the child's family, and any proposed treatment must be acceptable to the family. Parents are usually better agents of change than children, and treating parents and children together is more effective than treating children alone.

The mainstay of management is to aim for a balanced diet rather than a restrictive one, avoiding too many energy dense foods. An appointment with a dietician may be offered. Many parents find a traffic light system of green (can eat as often as wants), amber (mealtimes) and red (rare treat) helpful. A multifaceted approach to childhood obesity is favoured in the recent NICE guidelines.

Physical activity should be encouraged, but bear in mind that overenthusiastic exercise may expose a child's obesity, cause embarrassment and be abandoned. Walking and cycling are a good start. The psycho-social consequences of obesity may be the most important for a child.

Scenario 10

Mrs Littlejohn would like to discuss her 4-year-old son, John. He is smaller than other children at nursery and is a picky eater. Mrs Littlejohn is of average height.

According to popular general practice magazines, about 40% of parents worry about their child's eating. However, children with 'failure to thrive' have a weight below the 3rd centile for their age and a declining growth velocity and/or a drop across two or more centile lines on a growth chart. John needs to have serial measurements of height and weight to make such a diagnosis. *Note:* A reduced weight compared with a normal head circumference in a seemingly well child is a sign of reduced food intake. It is worth exploring a typical day's intake and suggesting keeping a food diary for a week. Consider offering a printed leaflet from a website such as Patient UK. You need to arrange follow-up and to see/examine John.

Consider: Short parents generally have short children. Children's growth pattern may also follow that of their parents (this is called constitutional delay). Other commoner causes which may be explored are:

- Psychosocial problems (are things happy at home?)
- Lactose or cow's milk protein intolerance (does he refuse or have any problems after any particular type of food?)

A brief history should be taken of whether John has tummy aches, longstanding (chronic is a word often misinterpreted as severe) diarrhoea, birth weight (small?) and other problems with feeding or health. Lactose intolerance may follow an acute gastrointestinal infection and may persist for months. Cow's milk protein intolerance is rare after the age of 2 years. Suggesting other types of milk or dietary change should not take place at the first consultation unless there is a clear indication.

Rarer causes to be borne in mind are: cystic fibrosis, coeliac disease, intrauterine growth restriction, chronic severe asthma and chronic urinary infections.

Note: Consider how to apply similar approach to a 12-month-old who is failing to gain weight, or a 1-month-old who is 'failing to gain weight' according to the parents.

Scenario 11

You are asked to see Jenny Smith, a 16-year-old schoolgirl with acne on her forehead, chin and back. Washing with coal tar soap smells 'awful and hasn't helped at all.' Advise her.

Introduce yourself and briefly recap, checking where she has spots (assessing severity) and exploring her ideas, concerns and expectations. Emphasize that this condition is extremely common in teenagers.

Are there any social pressures such as bullying or romantic frustration?

Has she complied with treatment so far? Explore her ideas on personal hygiene. There are many (commercially available) antiseptic soaps that are more pleasant than coal tar. She should try and avoid touching, scratching or 'popping' her spots if she wants to avoid scarring.

You would like to promote a healthy lifestyle and hygiene. However, it may be useful to dispel the myths that acne severity is related to bad diet or poor hygiene. There is no evidence to support this.

There are several approaches to treatment. Many GPs adopt a stepwise approach to treatment, with 2–3 months at each 'step'. The first step is soap and over-the-counter gels and lotions. The second step is topical treatments, such as benzoyl peroxide. This also comes in combination with topical erythromycin or clindamycin. Emphasize that oral antibiotics may appear to have 'cured her best friend overnight', but topical treatments should be tried first unless acne is very severe. Some GPs offer a topical retinoid, such as differin, further down the line, but this can have adverse effects such as photosensitivity and drying of the skin.

As a next step she could be treated with an antibiotic (erythromycin or tetracycline). It is worth mentioning that these also take time to work and can have side effects, such as (for tetracyclines) stomach upset, allergies and sensitivity to sunlight. If, however, an antibiotic is not effective within 3 months, she could (girls only) be prescribed Dianette in addition. You need to explain that Dianette is a contraceptive and may cause headache or breast tenderness. There is an increased risk of deep venous thrombosis. If acne disappears with antibiotics and/or Dianette, the antibiotics are weaned off, then the Dianette stopped, and the gel may be left as a prophylactic.

If all fails and she has bad acne, she may be asked if she would like to be referred to a 'skin specialist' to be assessed in clinic for other treatments which may have more side effects and are not started by GPs (e.g. roaccutane)

Printed information/advice for acne may be helpful. Agree on a plan and a sensible follow-up period.

Scenario 12

Mrs Sanders has come to discuss her 14-year-old daughter, Hermione. Hermione has, for over a year, been missing school on average once a week with terrible stomach aches. She has had numerous ultrasounds, blood tests and at one point a CT looking for appendicitis (these were all normal).

It is hard to distinguish functional abdominal pain from organic abdominal pain. Only the presence of alarm symptoms or signs increases the probability of an organic disorder and justifies further diagnostic testing:

- Involuntary weight loss
- Deceleration of linear growth
- Gastrointestinal blood loss
- Significant vomiting
- Chronic severe diarrhoea
- Unexplained fever
- Persistent right upper or right lower quadrant pain
- Family history of inflammatory bowel disease

Diagnostic triage to discriminate functional abdominal pain from organic disorders in young people aged 4–18 years with chronic abdominal pain can be carried out by a GP by means of assessment of alarm symptoms or signs and physical examination. Additional diagnostic evaluation is not required in children without alarm symptoms. Testing may be carried out to reassure children and their parents.

Treatment will have to take place over several consultations. If the condition suddenly deteriorates, she may need to be assessed in A&E.

- Deal with psychological factors
- Educate the family (an important part of treatment)

- Focus on return to normal functioning rather than on the complete disappearance of pain
- Best to prescribe drugs judiciously as part of a multifaceted, individualized approach, to relieve symptoms and disability
- For more information: International Foundation for Functional Gastrointestinal Disorders (www.aboutkidsgi.org/)

Scenario 13

Mrs Smith has come to discuss her son William, aged 6. He has always been an active boy and this sometimes caused difficulties at nursery. Now a primary school teacher has suggested that he might have attention-deficit hyperactivity disorder (ADHD). Please advise her.

GPs are often the first to be approached first by a concerned parent anxious to know if a poorly performing or badly behaved child has a developmental problem or needs extra help.

There is no biological marker (blood test or scan) which currently identifies children with ADHD. A GP is not in a position to diagnose ADHD – many of the behaviours associated with ADHD are seen in normal children! Screen for:

- **Inattention:** poor attention to detail and organization of tasks, appears not to listen, easily distracted, forgetful, lack of concentration on a given task
- **Impulsiveness:** Shouts out answers to questions, difficulty in taking turns or queuing, talks over others, lack of social awareness
- **Hyperactivity:** fidgets, does not stay in seat, inappropriate running or climbing

Diagnosis requires several such behaviours to be present in more than one setting (e.g. home and school) for > 6 months. Prior to further referrals it is accepted practice to request a hearing test. Sensitive inquiry into family and domestic circumstances may yield reasons for odd behaviour and this could be followed up in further consultations. You should also consider sensitive screening questions for autism, Asperger's syndrome and the autistic spectrum.

As with other childhood educational and development problems, if there are any clinical grounds or parental anxiety, then a referral may be made to child psychiatry or community paediatrics (this depends on local arrangements).

Scenario 14

Mrs Brown has come for the result of a CT scan, which was organized in a hurry when her daughter, Sophie, aged 3 was found to be ataxic and poorly coordinated at a visit for another problem. The CT shows 'a large posterior fossa lesion highly suggestive of an astrocytoma'.

There is no doubt that 5 minutes is not an appropriate length of time in which adequately to break this news. In reality the scan would have probably accompanied an urgent referral. Also, an in-depth knowledge of childhood cancers is not mandatory. The candidate would be expected to understand that extreme bad news is being given to a parent, and to break the bad news appropriately, establishing the parent's ideas, concerns and expectations at the outset. The candidate would also be expected to have a basic idea of what the next steps would involve.

Breaking bad news

- Ask the receptionist to hold your calls/indicate that this is so
- Introduce yourself to the mother.
- Is anyone else with her? Would she like them present?
- Recap on what has happened – a good way to establish ideas, concerns and expectations
- Offer the warning shot: 'The scan result is back, and I m afraid it s not good news'
- Break the bad news. Avoid using confusing or misleading words like 'lesion' or 'growth', especially if the likelihood is 'cancer' (this is unambiguous)
- Acknowledge that you have given her difficult news, ask if she understands what you have said and if she has any questions?
- You may have time to go on to 'what happens next', which is itself a likely question from the parent

Whilst a detailed knowledge of paediatric tumours is not essential, that of a broad approach to intracranial problems in children certainly is. Sophie can (if not already) be referred urgently to a 'brain specialist' and a 'children's cancer specialist' who will advise on the next steps. Tests that may need to be done include EEG, skull X-ray, CT and/or MRI scans, and blood tests. Treatment depends on these further tests and specialist advice, and may involve surgery or medication. Most importantly, you and the practice will continue to offer Sophie and her family support. A follow-up appointment should take place in the next few days; printed advice and contact details for a relevant self-help group may be valuable also.

Advice about a baby

Scenario 1

Mr White has come to see you following the birth of his daughter, Savannah, at 33 weeks' gestation. She needed some oxygen at birth and spent a week having tube-feeding in the Special Care Unit. Mr White would like to know what problems might lie in the future for her as a result.

Prematurity advice

There may be a large number of marks available for finding out Mr White's ideas, concerns and expectations, e.g.:

- She is so small and fragile, how should I hold her?
- Will she grow and be normal?
- Should we let the family visit?
- What should we do if she won't feed?
- How will I/we/her mother cope?
- Is she at risk of cot death?
- What should we do if we are worried about her?

Some of the issues you may wish to raise and explore may tally with the parental anxieties:

- **Feeding difficulties**: The suckling reflex develops between 32 and 36 weeks' gestation. Some babies will initially struggle with feeding, and may need smaller, more regular feeds or support with nasogastric feeding. As they are small they dehydrate easily, and fluid balance needs to be maintained
- Premature babies frequently have **gastro-oesophageal reflux** and sometimes an immature gag reflex (risk of aspiration). Some will need antireflux medication and follow-up with a speech and language therapist

- Small and premature babies are at increased risk of **low blood sugar** in the first few days, especially if they have feeding problems. Parents should seek advice if their child is excessively jittery
- Premature birth can be a difficult time for parents, and admission to hospital may interfere with the normal **bonding** between them and their new baby. Parents have difficulty dividing attention between the new baby and any older children. A sensitive question about how things are at home may yield some discussion
- Some premature babies are distressed at birth. Others are more prone to chest infections, bronchiolitis and other chest problems in infancy. Premature babies are also prone to apnoea attacks. Parents should be encouraged to get their child seen if they are worried about their child's breathing
- **Thermoregulation** (hypothermia) – premature babies have an immature temperature control system; it is very important that she is kept warm. Kangaroo care, skin-to-skin contact with the mother or father, is claimed to be effective in maintaining temperature and to help with parent–child bonding.
- **Jaundice** of prematurity: 80% of premature babies (see Chapter 6).
- Premature babies are more at risk of **infection** – reduced maternal antibodies in the womb and also if not breast fed. This includes chest infections, meningitis and necrotizing enterocolitis (increased risk in bottle-fed babies – necrotizing enterocolitis is also seen in roughly 10% of babies under 1500 g). Breast feeding should be encouraged in preference to bottle feeding in the absence of contraindications. 'Was mum told to avoid breast feeding for any reason?'
- She may need to be followed up regularly by the ophthalmologist during the first year. This is because sometimes the oxygen needed at birth can affect the blood vessels in the back of the eyes (**retinopathy of prematurity**). When this is severe, early laser surgery may prevent blindness
- Some premature babies are anaemic because their bone marrow is immature or because of the large number of blood tests that they have had in the special care unit. For this reason they are often given an **iron supplement** to take after leaving the special care unit. Late anaemia may also occur
- **Patent ductus arteriosus**: in some premature and full-term babies the ductus does not close. If the baby is breathless, sweaty, pale or blue when feeding, then an urgent opinion should be sought. This is usually picked up on the baby check as a heart murmur at birth or 6 weeks

- There is a slightly increased risk of cot death in premature babies (see advice below)

Conditions that are more common in very premature babies

- Intracranial haemorrhage (immature brain – blood vessels more fragile)
- Very low blood sugar
- Respiratory distress syndrome
- Chronic lung disease (where a child has been ventilated)
- Apnoeas
- Long term neurodevelopmental problems (follow-up needed)
- Deafness (especially if aminoglycoside antibiotics are needed)

Although parents are usually keen to find out as much as possible, the amount of information may be overwhelming.

Sources of support: Premature babies should be reviewed by a paediatrician in clinic and may, depending on their gestation and condition at birth, have a follow-up appointment for a hearing test and a review by an ophthalmologist. Sources of support are the midwife, health visitor and GP. For those who have been admitted to a special care baby unit or neonatal intensive care unit there should be a telephone number on the discharge letter which parents can ring for advice. There may be a premature baby group for informal support and advice and there are some very good websites such as www.bliss.org.uk.

Disabilities such as cerebral palsy, hearing loss, visual impairment and educational and developmental problems are associated with extreme prematurity. For most preterm infants of > 32 weeks' gestation, survival and longer term neurodevelopment are similar to those of infants born at term. Overall, outcomes are also good for infants born after shorter gestations. Most infants survive without substantial neurodevelopmental problems and most go on to attend mainstream schools, ultimately living independent lives.

Scenario 2

Mrs Evans has come in with her 3-week-old boy, Charles. Though she has breast fed thus far, she is finding it hard to keep up with his demands for feeds, and is tired. She also complains that her nipples are getting sore, and that she feels uncomfortable feeding Charles in public.

Should I breast feed?

It is appropriate to state that to examine the cracked nipple an appointment will need to be made with an appropriate chaperone present. Topical remedies such as nipple shields, Kamilosan or even some breast milk can be tried. If there is redness or swelling, topical or oral antibiotics may be needed but these will not harm the baby (oral penicillins are safe).

Advantages to breast feeding

- For the first month at least it confers some protection for baby against infection
- Less chance of allergy problems in baby
- Results in better bonding between mother and child
- Cheaper and possibly more convenient than bottle feeding
- Protects mother against breast and ovarian cancer
- Promotes weight loss
- Initially helps control postpartum bleeding

Working women often have problems breast feeding. Some employers are more supportive. It is possible to breast feed at home and express enough for the following day, but expressing milk and freezing it when mum is back at work can be tiring.

Scenario 3

The health visitor has asked you to see Mrs Arden. She and her husband lost their first child to cot death 3 years ago. Mrs Arden is anxious about the health of her new baby, Elizabeth, and has not been sleeping, even when Elizabeth is asleep, for fear that she stops breathing.

Cot death advice

Parents who have suffered a sudden and unexpected death of a baby often feel anxious when they have another baby. The Foundation for Sudden Infant Death has set up the Care of the Next Infant (CONI) programme to help parents work through some of their fears. CONI is run in hospitals and community health centres and involves midwives, paediatricians, GPs and health visitors. Through CONI, parents can:

- Receive weekly home visits by their health visitor, so they can talk freely about any worries and seek advice

- Keep a symptom diary to record their baby's health, which they can then discuss with their health visitor
- Monitor their baby's growth with a weight chart and weighing scales, to detect changes quickly
- Borrow apnoea (breathing) monitors which pick up movements as the baby breathes and will ring an alarm if movements stop for longer than 20 seconds
- Receive a room thermometer and guidance on bedding and clothing

Accepted advice for reducing the risk of cot-death:

- Avoid smoking in pregnancy (including passive smoking)
- Do not smoke in the same room as the baby
- Do not let the baby get too hot
- Keep the baby's head uncovered
- Place the baby on her back, with feet to the foot of the cot (prevents the baby wriggling under blankets) – as advocated by the 'Back to Sleep' campaign
- Keep cot in the parents' room for first 6 months
- Do not share bed with the baby if (either) parent is a smoker, has been drinking alcohol, has taken medication that causes drowsiness, or feels very tired
- It is dangerous to sleep together with the baby, whether in a bed or armchair
- If the baby is unwell, seek professional advice promptly (HV, GP, A&E, etc.)

Scenario 4

Miss Clare Wilcock has brought her 1-month-old girl, Ruby, to see you. She apparently has been vomiting after every feed for the last 2 weeks.

The standard advice about recapping and eliciting the mother's ideas, concerns and expectations applies here. You should express a wish to examine the baby.

Gastro-oesophageal reflux disease (GORD) is the commonest cause of vomiting in infancy. The vomiting may commence soon after birth but is more frequently delayed for a few weeks. The clinical features are:

- Vomiting usually occurs after a feed when a small amount of food is regurgitated. From then until the next feed regurgitation may continue
- At times the vomiting may be forceful and may even be 'projectile'
- Vomit is never bile-stained but may contain frank or altered blood or mucus. Bile-stained vomit implies a surgical cause – particularly volvulus – until proven otherwise

- Most infants with this condition thrive normally and are not distressed by it, although it can cause growth restriction
- There may be aspiration of milk – presents with cough and wheezing

Diagnosis is usually based on the clinical presentation. Differentials include: congenital hiatus hernia, gastroenteritis, pyloric stenosis and UTI.

Management involves:

1. Reassure: adequate winding, smaller, more frequent feeds. Raising the head of the crib has been shown to have no benefit. Usually resolves spontaneously by 12–18 months. It is recommended that babies who posset are laid on their backs (see cot death advice) to sleep
2. Thickened feeds, e.g. Carobel, SMA Staydown
3. Ranitidine and Gaviscon are licensed in infancy, Omeprazole and domperidone may be used but are unlicensed
4. Metoclopramide may help symptoms, but must be balanced against possible side effects

GORD complicated by failure to thrive should receive shared care between primary and secondary care. Surgery may be indicated if there is failure to thrive, oesophageal ulceration and recurrent or persistent aspiration.

Common causes of persistent vomiting in all age groups

- Posseting
- Overfeeding (a health visitor's input may help)
- Oesophageal reflux
- Pyloric stenosis (true projectile vomit in 2–6-week-olds)
- Chronic occult infection (e.g. urinary tract infection)
- Intermittent obstruction (e.g. malrotation or volvulus)
- Raised intracranial pressure (sudden/no nausea)
- Migraine (often with family history/headache/aura, etc.)
- Peptic ulcer (with upper abdominal pain)

Scenario 5

You have just performed a 6-week-check on Mrs Langdon's firstborn, James. You note that he has prominent epicanthal folds, low set ears and a single palmar crease. On listening to his heart, you can hear a pansystolic murmur. Discuss your findings with the mother.

The implication is a clinical suspicion that James has Down's syndrome, and it would be unfair to expect a candidate to cover every aspect of this diagnosis and its implications in 5 minutes. As ever, there are marks for ascertaining the parent's ideas, concerns and expectations. *Beware:* Feelings of intense disappointment, guilt, anger and denial may be elicited by such a diagnosis.

Do not forget to congratulate Mrs Langdon on her new baby. Look at the baby and refer to James by name. You are breaking the possibility of bad news (see p. 126 for a general approach). Whereas the majority of findings were entirely normal, a couple of things in the examination are of concern to you (the warning of possible bad news). 'These findings are sometimes associated with Down's syndrome. Do you have any experience of this condition?', is one way of breaking the news. Try and avoid bombarding the parent with information, and let them ask questions.

The diagnosis is not based purely on characteristic appearance. Clinical suspicion must be confirmed by a senior paediatrician. The blood test (for chromosome analysis) for the parents and the baby takes about a week to come back. It is in James's and his family's interests for his result to be known: for reassurance or for knowledge about the possible implications for James's health and wellbeing, and whether there is an increased risk of any future siblings being affected. There is also assistance and support available in the event of a positive diagnosis: from the practice, self-help groups and, if necessary, social support and benefits.

What happens next? Referral to an appropriate paediatrician, genetic counselling and chromosomal analysis blood tests should be the next steps. Remember that at this stage there is no firm diagnosis.

Implications of a diagnosis of Down's syndrome

- **Immediate/short term:** possible heart defects, duodenal atresia, developmental delay, possible low IQ (this varies – average 50), hearing and eyesight problems
- **Later medical complications:** increased risk of chest infections, hypothyroidism, early-onset Alzheimer disease, atlantoaxial instability and leukaemia
- However: life-expectancy and quality of life are constantly improving – and issues in the long term may be finding suitable employment and accommodation in adulthood.

Scenario 6

Miss Jayne Harvey has come to see you with her 8-week-old daughter, Samantha (asleep in her carry chair). 'Samantha has been crying for 2 days and is not herself. She cries until she is exhausted and then sleeps. My 3-year-old, Jason, was never like this...' Samantha is feeding well and she is making soft stools and wet nappies.

This station might also be raised in the exam as a focused history – in which case there may be a significant proportion of marks for the management plan. For guidance on how to manage such a scenario please refer to Chapter 5.

Scenarios to practise with colleagues (allow 5 minutes for each)

Scenario 1

You have been asked to see 12-year-old Anna and her mother by the practice nurse. Anna is thin and has had several chest and throat infections in the last year, each time requiring antibiotics. Your colleague who saw her at the last appointment suggested getting blood for a full blood count, fasting blood sugar and an erythrocyte sedimentation rate. Anna is scared of needles, and has refused to have the blood test, even with a topical anaesthetic.

Issues to consider:

- How to gain Anna's informed consent (vital clarification on consent issues can be obtained from the General Medical Council's '*0-18*' guidance)
- Establishing a rapport and the reasons why Anna is afraid
- Explaining to parent and child why the blood test will help
- Enlisting the mother's help to persuade Anna
- Asking Anna's mother if she is happy to hold her daughter's arm steady, or if she would like the practice nurse to

Scenario 2

Mrs Verity Cross is on the telephone angrily demanding to speak to a doctor. She brought her 12-month-old Joey in with a cold yesterday. One of your colleagues advised paracetamol on a 'dose by weight' basis. Instead of '20 mg/kg TDS' he advised '200 mg/kg TDS'. The mistake was spotted by a helpful pharmacist, who advised her to get back in touch with the surgery.

Issues to consider:

- How is Joey now? Offer to review him
- A sincere apology on behalf of the practice. However, you cannot comment on the circumstances as you were not there
- Dealing with an angry parent, avoid confrontation
- Offer an appointment with the doctor concerned
- Offer to talk to the practice team about preventing a mistake like this in future
- Offer to put Mrs Cross in contact with the practice manager if she would like to make a formal complaint

Further reading

Berger MY, Gieteling MJ, Benninga MA. Chronic abdominal pain in children. *BMJ* 2007;**334**:997–1002.

Bellman M, Kennedy N. *Paediatrics and Child Health: A Textbook for the DCH*. London: Churchill Livingstone, 2000: p. 139–41.

Collier J, Longmore M, Brinsden M. Raised intracranial pressure. In: *Oxford Handbook of Clinical Specialties*, 7th edn. Oxford: Oxford University Press, 2006: p. 200–1.

Colvin M, McGuire W, Fowlie PW. Neurodevelopmental outcomes after preterm birth. BMJ 2004;**329**:1390–3.

de Groot H, Brand PLP, Fokkens WF, Berger MY. Allergic rhinoconjunctivitis in children. *BMJ* 2007;**335**:985–8.

Edmunds L, Waters E, Elliott EJ. Evidence-based management of childhood obesity. *BMJ* 2001;**323**:916–9.

Evans JHC. Evidence based management of nocturnal enuresis. *BMJ* 2001;**323**:1167–9.

Gatrad AR, Sheikh A. 10-minute consultation: persistent crying in babies. *BMJ* 2004;**328**:330.

Gawkrodger DJ. *Dermatology: An Illustrated Colour Text*, 3rd edn. London: Churchill Livingstone, 2003: p. 32–3 (eczema).

General Medical Council. *0–18 Years: Guidance for All Doctors*. London: GMC, 2007.

Guevara JP, Stein MT. Evidence-based management of attention-deficit hyperactivity disorder. *BMJ* 2001:**323**:1232–5.

Harnden A, Shakespeare J. 10-minute consultation: MMR immunisation. *BMJ* 2001:**323**:32.

Huertas-Ceballos A. Common problems in preterm babies. In: Bellman M, Peile E, eds. *The Normal Child*. Edinburgh: Churchill Livingstone, 2006: p. 24–7.

Jamil T. Clinical casebook – four year old who is failing to thrive. *Pulse* Nov 2007.

Khot A, Polmear A. *Practical General Practice: Guidelines for effective clinical management*, 4th edn. London: Butterworth Heinemann, 2004: p. 84–5.

MacManus P, Iheanacho I. Don't use minocycline as first line oral antibiotic in acne. *BMJ* 2007;**334**:154.

Meremikwu M, Oyo-Ita A. Physical methods for treating fever in children. *Cochrane Database Syst Rev* 2003;(2):CD004264.

National Institute for Health and Clinical Excellence. *Feverish illness in children: Assessment and initial management in children younger than 5* years. London: NICE, 2007. www.nice.org.

National Institute for Health and Clinical Excellence. *Obesity: Guidance on the prevention, identification, assessment and management of overweight and obesity in adults and children. NICE clinical guideline 43*. London: NICE, 2006. www.nice.org.

O'Carroll N, Fitzsimons J, Carr S. 10-minute consultation: Asthma unresponsive to simple treatment in a child. *BMJ* 2008;**336**:447.

Papanikitas A, Bahal N, Chan M. *Get Through Clinical Finals: A Toolkit for OSCEs*. London: RSM Press, 2006: p. 13–4 (Breaking bad news), 128.

Sadleir LG, Scheffer IE. Clinical review: Febrile seizures. *BMJ* 2007;**334**: 307–11.

Sheikh A, Walker S. 10-minute consultation: Food allergy. *BMJ* 2002;**325**:1337.

Simon C, Everitt H, Kendrick T. *Oxford Handbook of General Practice*, 2nd edn. Oxford: Oxford University Press, 2005: p. 806, 808, 815, 898–901 (Summary of developmental and educational difficulties).

Townshend J, Hails S, McKean M. Clinical review: Management of asthma in children. *BMJ* 2007;**335**:253–7.

Wynne-Jones M. Should you act over teenager's drug misuse? *Pulse* Feb 2007.

Index

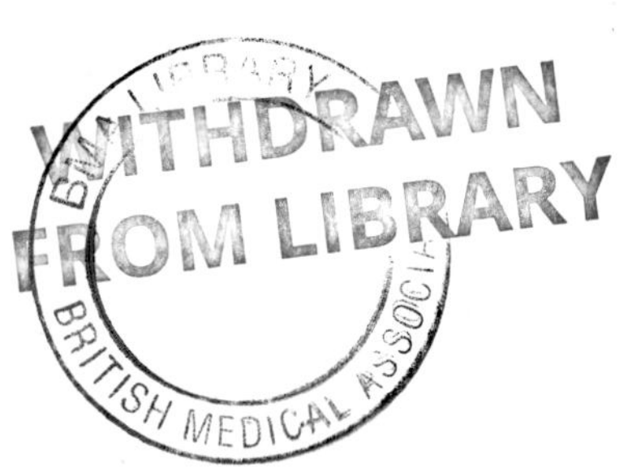
BMA LIBRARY
WITHDRAWN
FROM LIBRARY
BRITISH MEDICAL ASSOCIA